CONCISE GUIDE TO
Cross-Cultural Psychiatry

D1431821

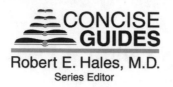

CONCISE
GUIDES

Robert E. Hales, M.D.
Series Editor

CONCISE GUIDE TO
Cross-Cultural Psychiatry

Albert C. Gaw, M.D.

Clinical Professor of Psychiatry
University of California–San Francisco

Medical Director for Long Term Care
Community Mental Health Services
Department of Public Health
City and County of San Francisco

Medical Director
San Francisco Mental Health Rehabilitation Facility
San Francisco General Hospital
Community Health Network of San Francisco
Department of Public Health
City and County of San Francisco

Lecturer on Psychiatry
Harvard Medical School

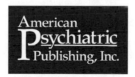

American Psychiatric Publishing, Inc.

Washington, DC
London, England

Manufactured in the United States of America on acid-free paper
04   03   02   01   4   3   2   1
First Edition

American Psychiatric Publishing, Inc.
1400 K Street, N.W.
Washington, DC 20005
www.appi.org

Library of Congress Cataloging-in-Publication Data
Gaw, Albert, 1939–
   Concise guide to cross-cultural psychiatry / Albert C. Gaw—1st ed.
      p. ; cm. — (Concise guides)
   Includes bibliographical references and index.
   ISBN 0–88048–907–3 (alk. paper)
      1. Psychiatry, Transcultural—Handbooks, manuals, etc.   2. Psychotherapy—
   Cross-cultural studies—Handbooks, manuals, etc.   3. Cultural psychiatry—Handbooks,
   manuals, etc.   4. Mental illness—Cross-cultural studies—Handbooks, manuals, etc.
   I. Title.   II. Concise guides (American Psychiatric Press)
      [DNLM: 1. Mental Disorders—ethnology.   2. Community Psychiatry.   3. Cross-Cultural
   Comparison.   4. Minority Groups—psychology.   WM 140 G284c 2001]
   RC455.4.E8 G39 2001
   616.89—dc21

                                                                                    00-050813
British Library Cataloguing in Publication Data
A CIP record is available from the British Library.

To my wife, Tina
and my daughter, Julie
and in loving memory of my mother, Chao H. Huang

CONTENTS

8 CULTURAL CONTEXT OF PSYCHOTHERAPY. 165

List of Tables

List of Figures

INTRODUCTION

to the Concise Guides Series

The Concise Guides Series from American Psychiatric Publishing, Inc., provides, in an accessible format, practical information for psychiatrists, psychiatry residents, and medical students working in a variety of treatment settings, such as inpatient psychiatry units, outpatient clinics, consultation-liaison services, and private office settings. The information in the Concise Guides is meant to complement the more detailed information to be found in lengthier psychiatry texts.

The Concise Guides address topics of special concern to psychiatrists in clinical practice. The books in this series contain a detailed table of contents, along with an index, tables, figures, and other charts for easy access. The books are designed to fit into a lab coat pocket or jacket pocket, which makes them a convenient source of information. References have been limited to those most relevant to the material presented.

Robert E. Hales, M.D., M.B.A.
Series Editor, Concise Guides

PREFACE

The *Concise Guide to Cross-Cultural Psychiatry* is a practical introductory guide for students and practitioners of mental health to address cultural issues in psychiatric care. The contents are derived from my experience in providing cross-cultural psychiatric service, teaching, and research in cross-cultural psychiatry for the past three decades. In this book, I attempt to weave cultural understanding into the biopsychosocial framework in psychiatric care.

With rapid changes in the demography of both the U.S. population and that worldwide, with advances in psychopharmacology, and with the revolutionary way in which mental health care is now delivered, practitioners in the field of mental health are increasingly challenged to provide psychiatric care to patients of different racial and ethnic backgrounds. This increasing cross-cultural encounter poses several key clinical issues: How does culture mold and influence the presentation of psychiatric symptoms? How are cultural issues woven into the *Diagnostic and Statistical Manual of Mental Disorders* (DSM-IV) used in psychiatric diagnoses? Is there racial and ethnic variation in the metabolism of psychotropic medications? What are the cultural factors that influence a patient's adherence or nonadherence to the taking of psychotropic medications? What is the cultural context of psychotherapy? How does the changing sociocultural context affect the clinician-patient relationship? How does one incorporate cultural concepts into clinical care?

To address these issues, I review pertinent findings from biological, psychological, sociological, and cultural factors and organize them into eight chapters, each addressing an important clinical area. Tables and figures are used to highlight key points in each chapter for easy reference in clinical situations and teaching. A glossary of terms is at the end of the book.

Acknowledgments I would like to thank Martin Lynds for help with manuscript preparation and the editorial staff at American

Psychiatric Publishing for editorial assistance. I also thank Steven K. Branch, M.D., Ph.D., and John A. Nichols, Psy.D., for their contributions to Chapters 6 and 7, respectively, and Francis Lu, M.D., for use of the *Annotated Bibliography on Cultural Psychiatry and Related Topics*. Carol Nadelson, M.D., Editor-in-Chief of American Psychiatric Publishing has been most encouraging and supportive. Finally, I thank my wife, Tina, for her understanding and good cheer as I pulled this volume together.

Albert C. Gaw, M.D.

CULTURE IN PSYCHIATRY

As our society becomes more diverse and the world evolves into a global village, the need to integrate culture into medicine and psychiatry becomes more critically important. Take the population of the United States as an example. If the current U.S. immigration pattern continues, by the mid-twenty-first century, the population of the United States will be approximately 53% Caucasian, 20% Hispanic, 16% African American, 10% Asian, and 1% other ethnic groups (1). Worldwide, increasing ease in international travel and migration and advances in information technology have enhanced interaction and intermingling of people from different cultural and social systems. As a result, practitioners of the health and mental health professions are increasingly being called on to treat patients from backgrounds very different from their own. Just how diverse the patient population can be is revealed by a cursory glimpse of the personal background of individuals treated in one day at the South Asian Clinic of the Cambridge Hospital in Cambridge, Massachusetts. Patients included an engineer from Nepal, a housewife from Indonesia whose marriage had been arranged through a mail-order advertisement, a housewife from India, and a student from China, among others.

Are Western-trained practitioners of physical and mental health well prepared to address the psychological distresses of individuals of varying cultural backgrounds? Can diagnosis and treatment be provided that will be perceived as relevant and acceptable by patients coming from backgrounds different from those of the clinicians?

Although modern psychiatry is grounded in both neuroscience and psychology, there have been recent efforts to enrich psychiatry by integrating into it various sociological and cultural materials (2). Understanding the *context* of the patient's experience is critical for enhancing greater precision in diagnosis and treatment. A clearer understanding of the concept of culture and its integration into medicine and psychiatry not only can increase clinicians' cultural sensitivity but also can sharpen their diagnostic acumen and aid in the formulation of treatment plans more congruent with the patient's cultural background.

In this chapter, I provide a brief overview of the development of various anthropological definitions of culture and summarize the essential elements of culture that are considered relevant to psychiatry. I propose adopting Ward Goodenough's definition of culture (see the next section in this chapter) as a clinically useful concept and propose examining how the application of such a concept can enrich psychiatric understanding and the work of mental health clinicians.

■ CONCEPTS OF CULTURE

Even among anthropologists, there is no consensus and consistency regarding the definition of the term *culture*. The purposes and the theoretical orientation of the authors frequently guide the definition of culture. In 1871, Sir Edward Burnett Tylor, a British anthropologist, penned what is generally accepted as the first clear and comprehensive definition of culture. He defined it as "that complex whole which includes knowledge, belief, art, law, morals, custom and any other capabilities and habits acquired by man as a member of society" (3, p. 1). Tylor's emphasis was on the *totality* of human achievements and that culture is *learned*. Since Tylor's time, definitions of culture have proliferated. Adopting a more pluralistic view of culture, Franz Boas considered that "culture embraces all the manifestations of social habits of a community, the reaction of the individual as affected by the habits of the group in which he lives, and the products of human activities as determined by these habits" (4). This interpretation of culture emphasizes *historicism,* that each community has its own autonomous world of *value* and *meaning,* and that culture *shapes* behavior. In 1952, Kroeber and Kluckholn attempted a critical review of concepts and definitions of culture and came up with 164 definitions (5). They summarized the central idea of culture formulated by most social scientists approximately as follows:

> Culture consists of patterns, explicit and implicit, of and for behavior acquired and transmitted by symbols, constituting the distinctive achievement of human groups, including their embodiments in artifacts; the essential core of culture consists of traditional (i.e., historically derived and selected) ideas and especially their attached values; culture systems may, on the one hand, be considered as products of action, on the other as conditioning elements of further action. (5, p. 357)

This definition emphasizes *patterns of and for* behavior, both *subjective* and *objective* legacies of human accomplishments, and that culture *impels* actions. They regarded culture not as a "force" acting within a group, but as an assumed "concreteness" created by individuals and by individuals operating as a group. It is internalized by individuals and by groups of individuals (5).

> Acts take place: (a) in time between persons, (b) in space in an environment partly made up of other persons. But because acts take place in time the past continues to influence the present. The history of the group leaves its precipitate—conveniently and by now, traditionally called "culture"—which is present in persons, shaping their perceptions of events, other persons, and the environing situation in ways not wholly determined by biology and by environmental press. Culture is an intervening variable between human "organism" and "environment." (5, p. 367–368)

Foreshadowing more contemporary definitions of culture that tend to separate the discrete acts of behavior from the values and beliefs that people use to interpret experience and generate behavior, Kroeber and Kluckhohn had this comment:

> Culture is not behavior nor the investigation of behavior in all its concrete completeness. Part of culture consists in norms for or standards of behavior. Still another part consists in ideologies justifying or rationalizing certain selected ways of behavior. Finally, every culture includes broad general principles of selectivity and ordering ("highest common factors") in terms of which patterns of and for and about behavior in very varied areas of culture content are reducible to parsimonious generalization. (5, p. 375)

Here, they called attention to the concept of culture as *standards of and for behavior and ideologies,* and the s*electivity* and *ordering* function of culture.

Geertz, commenting on the "thick description" of culture, leaned toward an interpretive theory of culture:

> The concept of culture I espouse . . . is essentially a semiotic one. Believing, with Max Weber, that man is an animal suspended in webs of significance he himself has spun, I take culture to be those webs, and the analysis of it to be therefore not an experiential science in search of law but an interpretive one in search of meanings. (6, p. 5)

Other more contemporary definitions of culture tend to distinguish more clearly between *actual* behavior on the one hand and the *abstract* values, beliefs, and perception of the world that lie behind that behavior on the other (7). The notion of culture as a set of standards that guides behavior assumes prominence. Havilan offered a modern definition of culture as follows:

> Culture is a set of rules or standards that, when acted upon by the members of a society, produce behavior that falls within a range of variance the members consider proper and acceptable. (7, p. 30)

Goodenough, a proponent of ethnoscience, equated culture with cognition, providing systems of classification that structure our understanding of the social and natural world (8). Goodenough formulated culture as

> a set of standards that taken as a guide for acting and interpreting the acts of others, leads to behavior the community's members perceive as in accord with their expectations of one another. (9)

Harwood, expanding on the concept Goodenough proposed, stated that

> By culture anthropologists and other social scientists generally mean standards for behavior that one acquires as a member of a social group. The standards include percepts, concepts, beliefs, and values that help individuals to order and thereby give meaning to their experience of both social relations and the physical world. (10, p. 27)

Anthropologist Hughes, who has written extensively on culture and psychiatry, defined culture as

> a construct that captures a socially transmitted system of ideas—ideas that shape behavior, categorize perceptions, and (through language) give names and thereby a putative reality to selected aspects of experience. As such, culture is a learned configuration of images and other symbolic elements (such as language) widely shared among members of a given society or social group which, for individuals, function as an orientational framework for behavior; and, for the group, serves as the communicational matrix which tends to coordinate and sanction behavior. . . . Cultural process is the mechanism for conveying values through and across generations. As such, it lays a complex web of meanings, purposes, and ultimate ends across the continuous stream of human experience and perception. (11, p. 7)

Hughes emphasized the *linguistic* aspect and *transmissibility* of culture across generations.

Finally, Kleinman, a psychiatrist and medical anthropologist, wrote a more contemporary definition of culture. He emphasized the *social* locus of culture:

> Culture is constituted by, and in turn constitutes, local worlds of everyday experience. That is to say, culture is built up ("realized") out of the everyday patterns of daily life activities—common sense, communication with others, and the routine rhythms and rituals of community life that are taken for granted—which reciprocally reflect the patterning downward of social relations by shared symbolic apparatuses—language, aesthetic sensibility, and the core value orientations conveyed by master metaphors. In these local worlds, experience is an important flow of communication, interaction, and negotiation—that is, it is social, not individual—which centers on agreement and contestation about what is most at stake and how that which is at stake, is to be sought and gained. Gender, age cohort, social role and status, and personal desire all inflect this small moral universe in different ways. The upshot is culture in the making, in the process that generate action and that justify practices. Thus, the locus of culture is not the mind of the isolated person, but the interconnected body/self of groups: families, work settings, networks, whole communities. (12, p. 16)

Considering the various definitions of culture that potentially can be applied to psychiatry, the National Institute of Mental Health (NIMH) Culture and Diagnosis Group, which provided cultural variables to the American Psychiatric Association's *Diagnostic and Statistical Manual of Mental Disorders,* fourth edition (DSM-IV) (13), came up with a more clinically oriented definition of culture:

> Meanings, values, and behavioral norms that are learned and transmitted in the dominant society and within its social groups. Culture powerfully influences cognitions, feelings, and the "self" concept, as well as the diagnostic process and treatment decisions. (14)

This definition of culture incorporates some of the key concepts from cultural anthropology reviewed earlier. It encompasses both psychosocial and intrapsychic phenomenon. It reflects a clinical orientation more consistent with the tasks of psychiatry and clinicians. It subsumes biological, psychological, and cultural variables operating in a web of social network.

■ ESSENTIAL FEATURES OF CULTURE

The essential features of culture are summarized in Table 1–1 and described in more detail below.

Culture is learned. Humans learned culture (7). Unlike biological endowment, learned behavior constitutes the essential component of culture. It includes people's assumptions about life. Culture consists of the ideals, values, and assumptions about life that are widely shared and that guide specific behaviors. Culture is a collective creation. It is socially constructed by human beings in interaction with others.

Culture refers to systems of meanings. Culture refers to systems of meanings through what Geertz calls "webs of significance," which govern the conduct and understanding of people's lives (6). These systems are distinguished from society itself in that the term *society* generally refers to the community of people. Meaning systems consist of negotiated agreements such as the relationship between a word, behavior, or other symbol and its corresponding significance or meanings (6).

TABLE 1–1. **Essential components of culture**

Culture is learned.

Culture refers to systems of meanings.

Culture acts as a shaping template.

Culture is taught and reproduced.

Culture exists in a constant state of change.

Culture includes patterns of both subjective and objective components of human behavior.

Culture acts as a shaping template and as a body of learned behaviors. Culture, as a body of learned behaviors common to a given human society, acts rather like a template, with predictable form and content, for shaping behavior and consciousness within a human society from generation to generation (5).

Culture is taught and reproduced. In a manner parallel to that of genes, culture is transmitted across generations through family and human institutions (7). Concepts, values, beliefs, mores, and systems of meanings essential for human survival as a group are transmitted across generations.

Culture exists in a constant state of change. As such, culture is relativistic; different societies agree on different relationships and meanings at different points in time and space (7).

Culture includes patterns of both the subjective and the objective components of human behavior. The domain of culture includes both patterns of the symbolic phenomena of the mental apparatus (central nervous system and mind) and the objective, observable aspects of human behavior and interaction. Anthropologists refer to these, respectively, as *implicit* and *explicit* patterns of behavior (5), or the *ideational* and the *phenomenal order of reality* (9).

■ IDEATIONAL ORDER OF REALITY OF CULTURE

The anthropologist Goodenough recognized two related orders of reality about culture:

1. *Objective culture.* The "phenomenal order of observed events and the regularities they exhibit . . . [are] a property of the community as a material system of people, their surroundings, and their behavior" (9).
2. *Subjective culture.* "Ideational order is non-material, being composed of ideal forms as they exist in people's minds, propositions about their interrelationships, preference ratings regarding them, and recipes for their mutual ordering as means to desired ends" (9).

Because the functions of the brain and its mental apparatus are a primary concern of psychiatry, understanding of the ideational order of culture is directly relevant to psychiatry. Culture provides the understanding of the experience of people in states of health and illness. Culture patterns the expression of psychic distress into symptoms generally regarded as "mental illness." Culture influences the procedures that are transacted between the "sufferers" and "healers" in the process of diagnosis and cure. Moreover, because culture encompasses ideational aspects of human behavior, it is essential that we understand how culture is operationalized in the mind.

Goodenough considered ideational order to consist of

> standards for deciding what is, standards for deciding what can be, standards for deciding how one feels about it, standards for deciding what to do about it, and standards for deciding how to go about doing it. People use their standards as guides for all the decisions, little as well as big, which they must make in the course of everyday life. As the members of a community go about their affairs, constantly making decisions in the light of their standards, the pattern characterizing the community as a whole are brought into being and maintained. (9)

In short, "culture is a set of standards for behavior which a group of people attribute to those around them and which they used to orient their own behavior" (10).

As is further elaborated below, this definition of culture has both heuristic and clinical applicability in both medicine and psychiatry. By examining the different components of culture, we can draw application for the understanding the *context* (culture background) of the behavior of the patient. Furthermore, because the clinical practice setting encompasses groups of professionals and other people operating in a social network, decisions based on implicit and explicit standards for individual and group behavior are made all the time, and their results guide the actions of clinicians. An understanding of the standards for behavior that subculture provides for a clinical setting can be useful to both students and professionals in such systems for accomplishing desired tasks and goals. Thus, besides being a useful clinical tool for understanding individual patients, I believe the concept of culture can be equally useful as a tool for system analysis.

■ COMPONENTS OF CULTURE AS APPLIED TO CLINICAL CARE

An examination of the operation of the *components* of culture in clinical care can further enhance understanding of the utility of the concept of culture in medicine and psychiatry.

Percepts and Concepts

A *percept* is "an impression in the mind of something perceived by the senses, viewed as the basic component in the formation of concepts" (15). Percepts are the building blocks for concepts in the brain and mental apparatus. *Concept,* on the other hand, is "a general idea or understanding, especially one derived from specific occurrences" (15).

Sensory impressions conveyed to the higher centers of the brain are subjected to the cognitive interpretive processes of the individual's experiences that give meanings to these impressions. Concepts are then formed and are usually encoded in words. Words such as *family, patriotism, anxiety,* and *schizophrenia* are examples of concepts that convey a certain meaning. By transforming sensory experiences of the phenomena around us into percepts and concepts, human beings can begin to make sense of what *is* in the environment and can communicate their experiences. Thus, percepts and concepts are important because they tell us what the world *is.*

Let us consider the Korean concept of *hwa-byung* and its relation to the Korean culture. The word *hwa* means "fire" or "anger," and *byung* means "illness." Literally translated, *hwa-byung* is an illness of anger. *Hwa-byung* describes a cluster of symptoms consisting of mixed depressive and anxiety disorders, with characteristic symptoms of a feeling of mass or heaviness and oppression in the chest or abdomen. It is thought to be a unique Korean culture-bound syndrome. Feelings of *haan* are thought to contribute to *hwa-byung* (16). *Haan,* in turn, refers to

> an individual and collective subconscious emotional complex among Korean people, involving suppressed feelings of anger, rage, despair, frustration, holding grudges, indignation, and revenge. It is a syndrome believed to result from victimization of a Korean person both as an individual and as a Korean, and is thought to be an important contributing factor to the development of *hwa-byung* ("anger disease"). (16, p. 595)

What is interesting about the *hwa-byung* phenomenon is that when extreme anger and sorrow are suppressed, the feelings can manifest as a series of somatic complaints, including an "abdominal mass." Although the patient may not necessarily label it as a psychosomatic illness, Korean people clearly understand the psychogenic aspect of the concept of *hwa-byung*. In other words, although the manifestation of the complaints is clearly somatic in nature, Korean people recognize that the origin of the conflict is centered in the mind and the mental apparatus. When put this way, the Korean people, cognizant of their historical and long social suffering, capture the collective anger of their social experience of oppression in *hwa-byung*. Here we see how a social and historical experience precipitates as patterned behaviors that are expressed as a psychosomatic phenomenon.

Propositions

Propositions are ways in which percepts and concepts can be related to one another. Simply having percepts and concepts is not enough. The mind must be able to manipulate these symbols so that the relationships of things around us can be understood. We need to know how things, events, and people are related. Proposition allows us to correlate the relationships between percepts and concepts in three ways:

- *Locational.* A proposition that suggests a geographic or locational relationship. For example, in clinical medicine, a key characteristic of the concept of appendicitis is the presence of a rebound tenderness located at the right lower quadrant of the abdomen. (Besides rebound tenderness, other symptoms of appendicitis include pain, fever, and vomiting, which suggest the inflammation of the vermiform appendix). Tenderness located at the lower right quadrant of the abdomen conveys a locational relationship. Inferences made about the relationship of pain and its associated symptoms in that particular bodily location form an important basis upon which the physician makes the diagnosis of appendicitis.

- *Part/whole.* A proposition that links the relationship of the concept to a larger "whole." This is similar to the idea of *figure/ground* in psychology. For example, in psychiatry, early morning awakening as a feature of sleep disturbance suggests depression. (Besides sleep disturbances, other symptoms of depression include a subjective feeling of being "down," social withdrawal, loss of interest, increased feeling of guilt, weight loss, diminished energy level, helplessness, hopelessness, loss of concentration, and the emergence of suicidal thoughts.) The diagnosis of depression is suggested because early morning awakening is *part* of a *whole* syndrome of depression.

- *Causal.* Concepts that are related in a cause-and-effect manner. Consider the hypothesis of the Freudian notion that introjected aggression leads to depression. Certain individuals experience depression because of difficulty managing anger and aggression. A cause-and-effect relationship between aggression and depression is implied in this hypothesis. This concept has guided the psychotherapeutic principle of encouraging patients to ventilate their feelings as if to rid the body of noxious psychological substances. It is presumed that when anger is expressed outwardly in a socially acceptable manner instead of directed toward the self, a therapeutic effect that relieves depression can occur.

Beliefs

Beliefs are propositions considered to be true. Certain individuals hold beliefs that are contrary to the realities experienced by others around them, cannot be corrected by reason, and are beyond the realm of acceptable social behavior. There are also ego-syntonic beliefs in the context of the clinical setting that do not fit into cultural norms; these would be labeled *delusional*. At the hospital in which I worked, there was a woman who regularly described herself as a member of the "holy family" every Christmastime. She considered herself to be the Holy Mother, her son to be Jesus, and her boyfriend to be Joseph, the father of Jesus. No amount of logical reasoning could dissuade her from this belief.

Values

Values suggest concepts and propositions organized into a hierarchy of preferences. Values are important principles that guide priorities in the distribution of resources. If health care personnel value sustaining life more than preparation for death, their actions and allocation of resources will be guided accordingly. Values also guide behaviors. The differences in values that influence the behavior differences between Oriental and Western culture—in this case, American culture versus Japanese culture—are depicted in Table 1–2.

Operational Procedures, or Recipes

Operational procedures, or recipes, are ways in which people organize their effort to accomplish certain tasks. Procedures guide actions. We are guided daily by "habits" that routinely get us through the day. In an educational setting, students and trainees are taught procedures regarding how to do a physical or a mental status examination, to diagnose a disease or an illness, to prescribe drugs, or to perform psychotherapy or surgery. In short, the learning of procedures allows us to get things done and to accomplish certain goals.

TABLE 1–2. **Comparison of cultural values and traditions between American and Japanese civilization**

American civilization	Japanese civilization
Individualism	Familism
Independence	Interdependence
Protestant ethic: emphasis on work, science and technology; human ability to control the environment; religious support of human endeavors toward economic and material progress	Confucian ethics: loyalty between lord and subordinates; intimacy between father and sons; propriety between husband and wife; order between elder and junior; trust between friends
Present and future orientation	Past, present, and future orientation
Tolerance of differences	Tolerance for similarities
Emphasis on self-fulfillment, self-development	Emphasis on interpersonal relationships
Emphasis on individual achievement	Emphasis on group achievement
Emphasis on newness	Emphasis on newness and change in the context of tradition

Source. Reprinted from Yamamoto J: Consideration of creativity in Japan. *Scientific Bulletin* 7(2):84–87, 1982, pp. 84–85.

Culture Versus Subculture

Culture involves very broad guidelines or standards governing behavior in a wide variety of contexts, from cradle to grave. When narrower sets of standards, which govern how one acts in a smaller range of behavior with a particular set of actors, are used, we refer these standards for behavior as a *subculture* (10). The biomedical profession can be regarded as a subculture in that it has its own percepts, concepts, propositions, beliefs, values, and operating procedures. As members of a subcultural group of a professional society, clinicians' behaviors are markedly influenced by those sets of standards for behavior held by that subcultural group.

Operating Culture

At any one time, a person can possess different sets of standards for behavior—as though the mind simultaneously holds several types of behavioral software. The standards a person uses at a particular time and place with significant others are referred to as an *operating culture.*

Ethnicity

Closely related to the concept of culture but applied to a narrower focus is *ethnicity.* The sociologist Schermerhorn defined an ethnic group as "a *collectivity* within a larger society having a real or putative common ancestry, memories of a shared historical past, and a cultural focus on one or more symbolic elements defined as the epitome of their peoplehood" (17). Irish, Jews, Chinese, African Americans, and Hispanics are all ethnic concepts. Thus, ethnicity defines collectivities on the basis of both common origins and shared symbols and standards for behavior (culture), and these collectivities are embedded in a larger social system (10).

Harwood listed several reasons as to how understanding ethnicity in health care can improve quality:

- By removing class and professional barriers to the realization of ethnically appropriate health care
- By eliciting the patient's model of the problem and treating the illness that is congruent with the patient's belief system
- By making medical treatment more conformable with the patient's lifestyle
- By improving the articulation between mainstream and non-mainstream sources of health care (10)

■ IMPLICATIONS OF THE CONCEPT OF CULTURE IN CLINICAL CARE

How does an understanding of the concept of culture enhance clinical psychiatry?

1. *It enhances diagnosis and treatment.* Leighton reminded us of the common ground between cultural anthropology and clinical psychiatry:

   > Shared values, shared perceptions of reality, and shared symbols by which thinking and interpersonal relationships are conducted constitute an interesting common ground between cultural anthropology and clinical psychiatry. Understanding a patient's feeling and values, perceptions of reality, and use of symbols is essential in diagnosis and treatment. When there is a cultural difference between patient and clinicians it behooves the latter to grasp something about the culture in question and about culture as both a social and psychological process. (18, p. 211)

   Values, orientations, and customs provide the necessary framework for comprehending an individual's particular mix of personality and the social-environmental influences. An understanding of culture guides the clinician to choose the right questions to ask, to interpret the responses, and to lay out a therapeutic plan and case-management plan that is congruent with the relevant factors at work in a patient's life (18).

2. *It fosters clinicians' sensitivity toward patients.* Just as the handling of countertransference issues stemming from the background of the psychotherapist during the therapeutic encounter would require careful analysis, cultural bias toward patients may be reduced through systematic inquiry into the cultural reactions of the clinician. Hughes (11) provided an outline of such an inquiry:

   - What about this patient's appearance or behavior makes me *think* what I am seeing and hearing is pathology?
   - What are the sources of the putative "pathologic" characterization?
   - What label(s) am *I* subconsciously applying to this patient, and where did they come from?
   - What social class or group am I *assuming* the patient belongs to, and what do I know about that? What are my own

prejudices about that group, and where do such characterizations come from—childhood directives and role-modeling, family inculcated out-group attitudes, scanning of current events that may reinforce preexisting stereotypes?

- Other than "pathology," what other hypotheses come to mind to explain this unusual behavior and/or mentation?
- What other label could I use to describe this behavior instead of pathology?
- What are the circumstances of the *referral* (if a referral), and what is the descriptive *spoken* language used by other health care providers in conveying information about the patient?
- What labels and summary inferences are used in the patient's *chart* or in the referral? How many of the empirical observations such as labels purport to reflect can I recreate from the written record (knowing that a medical record needs to be highly selective in the amount of data reported)? What do I know about the person or persons making such comments in the record?

3. *It enriches psychiatric knowledge.* Foulk (19) mentioned several areas in which a clinically useful definition of culture can enrich psychiatric knowledge:

- How people think, behave, and feel
- How children are raised, how and by whom, and how they acquire rules for behavior
- How personality is formed, including one's sense of self, personal psychology, and *self-esteem* [italics added]
- What the standards and values are one uses to evaluate others and guide one's behavior, including guidelines for diagnosing mental illness, ways of expression of emotional distress and their coping, and in prescribing treatments

4. *It provides guidelines for judgment of "normality" versus "abnormality" of behavior.* The act of diagnosis, in a way, is an

interpretation of the meaning of a cluster of behaviors according to a cultural norm. Whether the diagnosis indicates normal or abnormal behaviors will depend on the deviation from the standards of the norm that the diagnostician used at the time. It behooves clinicians to learn the standards from the perspective of the patients regarding the determination of deviancy when labeling aberrant behaviors as "mental disorders" so that misjudgments will not be made.

5. *It provides a proper understanding of human beings, whether their behavior is normative or deviant.* Culture is not just idiosyncratic behavior influenced by one's genetic endowment, it is formed primarily during the process of socialization from infancy to adulthood. We are inculcated with cultural concepts that are embedded into the fabric of our central nervous system and mental apparatus. Culture is intimately related to and expressed through our personality. At any particular moment in time and setting, culture provides the standards, or rules, for behavior. During their operation, whether conscious or unconscious, cultural concepts serve as an informational system that signals to the individual what is in the world and what proper procedures to take under specific circumstances to accomplish desired goals.

Culture *constructs* illness experiences and shapes their expression through its conventional *idiom*. As Kleinman et al. pointed out,

illness represents personal, interpersonal, and cultural reactions to disease or discomfort. Illness is shaped by cultural factors governing perception, labeling, explanation, and valuation of the discomforting experience, processes embedded in a complex family, social and cultural nexus. Because illness experience is an intimate part of social systems of meaning and rules of behavior, it is strongly influenced by culture: it is as we shall see, culturally constructed. (20)

Understanding of the *context* of the illness experience is essential in making clinical judgments. Culture provides the essential *context* for such critical analysis.

■ CONCLUSION

It is hoped that this review of the anthropological concept of culture and this clinically oriented definition of culture will sharpen the clinician's diagnostic judgment, correlate the context of cultural background in the patient's experience of illness, and provide cultural guidelines for the prescription of appropriate therapies and treatment. Integration of cultural concepts into medicine and psychiatry should enrich the clinician's understanding of patients in the clinical encounter. A paradigm that integrates culture into the biopsychosocial model of care should foster a holistic understanding of health and illness.

■ REFERENCES

1. U.S. Bureau of the Census: Percent distribution of population, by race and Hispanic origin: 1990, 2000, 2025, and 2050, in Current Population Reports. Washington, DC, U.S. Government Printing Office, 1992, pp 25–1095
2. Favazza AR, Oman M: Overview: foundations of cultural psychiatry, in Culture and Psychopathology. Edited by Mezzich JE, Berganza CE. New York, Columbia University Press, 1984, pp 15–35
3. Tylor E: Primitive Culture, Vol 1. Boston, Estes and Lauriat, 1874
4. Boas F: Summary of the work of the committee in British Columbia, in A Franz Boas Reader: The Shaping of American Anthropology, 1883–1911. Edited by Stocking G. Chicago, IL, University of Chicago Press, 1982
5. Kroeber AL, Kluckholn C: Culture: A Critical Review of Concepts and Definitions. Papers of the Peabody Museum of

American Archaeology and Ethnology, Harvard University. Cambridge, MA, Harvard University Museum, 1952

6. Geertz C: The Interpretation of Cultures. New York, Basic Books, 1973

7. Haviland WA: Cultural Anthropology, 6th Edition. New York, Holt, Rinehart, and Winston, 1990

8. Winthrop RH: Dictionary of Concepts in Cultural Anthropology. New York, Greenwood Press, 1991

9. Goodenough WH: Comments on cultural revolution. Daedalus 90:521–528, 1961

10. Harwood A (ed): Ethnicity and Medical Care. Cambridge, MA, Harvard University Press, 1981

11. Hughes CC: Culture in clinical psychiatry, in Culture, Ethnicity, and Mental Illness. Edited by Gaw AC. Washington, DC, American Psychiatric Press, 1992, pp 1–41

12. Kleinman A: How is culture important for DSM-IV? in Culture and Psychiatric Diagnosis: A DSM-IV Perspective. Edited by Mezzich JE, Kleinman A, Fabrega Jr H, et al. Washington, DC, American Psychiatric Press, 1996, pp 15–25

13. American Psychiatric Association: Diagnostic and Statistical Manual of Mental Disorders, 4th Edition. Washington, DC, American Psychiatric Association, 1994

14. Mezzich JE, Kleinman A, Fabrega L, et al (eds): Revised Cultural Proposals for DSM-IV (technical report). Pittsburgh, PA, NIMH Culture and Diagnostic Group, September, 1993

15. Morris W (ed): The American Heritage Dictionary of the English Language. New York, American Heritage Publishing Company, 1970

16. Kim LIC: Psychiatric care of Korean Americans, in Culture, Ethnicity and Mental Illness. Edited by Gaw AC. Washington, DC, American Psychiatric Press, 1993, p 347–375

17. Schermerhorn RA: Comparative Ethnic Relations: A Framework for Theory and Research. Chicago, IL, University of Chicago Press, 1970

18. Leighton AH: Relevant generic issues, in Cross-Cultural Psychiatry. Edited by Gaw AC. Boston, MA, John Wright-PSG, 1982, pp 199–236

19. Foulks EF: Discussion: relevant generic issues, in Cross-Cultural Psychiatry. Edited by Gaw AC. Boston, MA, John Wright-PSG, 1982, pp 237–246
20. Kleinman A, Eisenberg L, Good B: Culture, illness, and care, clinical lessons from anthropological and cross-cultural research. Ann Intern Med 88(2):251–258, 1978

■ RECOMMENDED FURTHER READING

For further information, please refer to Appendix B, Annotated Bibliography on Cultural Psychiatry and Related Topics.

2

CULTURAL INFLUENCES IN PSYCHIATRIC CARE OF NATIVE AMERICANS
A Paradigm

Given the ubiquitous influence of culture, how does a clinician go about mapping the domain of cultural information that will be useful in psychiatric care when faced with a patient whose ethnic background is different from that of the clinician? I propose using ethnicity as a central organizing principle to integrate cultural factors in psychiatric care. As noted in Chapter 1, Culture in Psychiatry, the concept of ethnicity is closely related to culture but differs from it in that it has a narrower focus. Schermerhorn (1) defined *ethnic group* as a "*collectivity* within a larger society having a real or putative common ancestry, memories of a shared historical past, and a cultural focus on one or more symbolic elements defined as the epitome of their peoplehood" (see Chapter 1, Culture in Psychiatry). Ethnic groups are usually bound by their common language, customs, traditions, and unique ways of living. Thus, the Irish have their shamrock and Saint Patrick's Day, the Chinese their August Moon Festival, and the Americans their Thanksgiving day.

Ethnic groups also have developed unique patterns of dealing and coping with mental distresses and illnesses (2–4). Ethnic concepts, values, and beliefs influence the way mental symptoms are expressed in individuals within the group. Ethnic standards provide the yardstick for defining whether certain behavioral patterns within that group are considered "normal" or "abnormal." Patterns of coping with mental distress for individuals and their families also vary with different ethnic groups. Thus, as the members of each group set about their daily activities, certain discernible patterns of health-seeking behaviors that characterized illness episodes continuously guide and influence them in moments of stress (2–4).

To illustrate the clinical utility of ethnicity, I select as a paradigm the cultural issues attending the psychiatric care of Native Americans. I choose Native Americans for three reasons. First, of the four major federally identified minority groups in the United States (Asian, African American, Hispanic, and Native American), I consider Native Americans to be the least understood. Although native to North America, they are frequently ignored and have been exploited. Second, Native Americans have been the object of intensive medical and anthropological studies. Thus, a rich body of literature on the culture of these native people is available for integration into the understanding of their health care. Third, the sharp contrast of Native American culture with that of the mainstream of the United States lends itself more easily to comparative study. My hope is that through the study of the cultural influence of psychiatric care for Native Americans, such a paradigm can be applied to the study of other cultural groups as well.

I propose that clinicians compile the following information to aid in examining cultural issues during psychiatric care of patients whose ethnic backgrounds diverge from that of the clinician (refer also to Chapter 5, Cultural Formulation, for a systematic examination of cultural information in psychiatric care). The list is not exhaustive but serves as a practical starting point that pulls together key cultural information regarding the conceptualization of the cultural context when delivering care to patients with such backgrounds.

1. Brief historical background for immigrant groups; include history of the group in country of origin, immigration experience, cultural values, pertinent demography, and psychiatric epidemiology

2. Health beliefs and cultural conceptions of mental health and illness, including stigma of mental illness
3. Expression of mental illness, including culture-bound syndromes
4. Family response to mental illness
5. Culturally congruent treatment measures

■ HISTORICAL BACKGROUND OF NATIVE AMERICANS

The terms *Native American, Indian,* and *American Indian* are used interchangeably in this chapter and refer to both the aboriginal people of North America and native Hawaiians. Evidence on the origin of the native people in North America remains inconclusive. It is generally believed that the first Native Americans migrated from Asia over the Bering Strait land bridge during the last Ice Age (5). The arrival of Columbus in 1492 in the Americas divides the history of the Indian people into the "pre-Columbian," or "precontact," and "post-Columbian," or "postcontact," periods. During the precontact period, Indians practiced farming in two large geographic areas: along the Rocky Mountains, and in the eastern half of the United States from the Gulf of Mexico to Canada (5). Early tribal medical beliefs seemed also to reflect where the Indians were located: the beliefs of those in the areas along the Rocky Mountains were quite similar to those of their Siberian ancestors; the beliefs of those along the eastern seaboard appeared closer to those of Europeans (6). Significant events in the recent history of American Indians are depicted in Table 2–1.

Several historical experiences that deprived Indian people of their cultural and ethnic identities are worth mentioning.

* *The conquest of the New World by European immigrants.* Through usurpation of land, pushing Indians into bloody tribal conflicts, exposure to Old World diseases such as smallpox, introduction of the corrupting influence of alcohol, and the results of starvation and malnutrition, the once teeming Native

TABLE 2–1. **American Indians and Alaska Natives: significant dates and periods in recent history**

Year(s)	Periods and events
Before 1492	Precontact period began at least 20,000 years ago. Approximately 300 tribal groups with many subdivisions within tribal groups. Indian peoples of the Americas spoke more than 1,000 unique languages, derived from 56 language families.
1492–mid-1800s	Some early contacts between American Indians and Europeans were positive, but these were the exception. Exploitation of Indians and their lands shaped the Indian/European relationship from the beginning of contact. The introduction of alcohol was used to take advantage of American Indians (e.g., in order to more easily "buy" land—a concept that was very foreign to Indians).
1500–1890	Epidemic era. Whites brought infectious diseases for which Indian people were not prepared immunologically. Five-sixths of some populations were killed by early epidemics. Leaders and other elders also died, leaving many communities without leadership. Also known as the Manifest Destiny era, a term coined in the mid-1800s to describe the desire of many Americans to possess a country that was larger than Europe and reached from coast to coast, led to destruction of American Indians, not only by epidemics and alcohol, but also by war, massive forced migrations, and the formation of reservations. Forced suppression of American Indian cultures and religions and education of children to be "white" also were important factors.
Early 1800s	The Bureau of Indian Affairs (BIA), a portion of the War Department, took responsibility for Indian health care.
Late 1800s	Revitalization movement. Religious movements were begun by American Indian people to try to regain lost culture. Heavily influenced by Christianity but with many traditional Indian practices.

(continued)

TABLE 2–1. **American Indians and Alaska Natives: significant dates and periods in recent history** (continued)

Year(s)	Periods and events
1849	The BIA, along with Indian health care, became part of the Interior Department.
1887	The Daws Act stipulated that communally owned (Indian) lands be divided into individual "allotments" of land to own and farm. As was the case many times before, much of this land found its way into white hands, often by fraud.
1890–1970	Assimilation era. Following the Wounded Knee massacre (1890), depression, alcoholism, and violence had reached their peaks on reservations. The overt extermination policy of the United States changed to a more subtle one of "assimilating" Indians into white culture. Many Indians agreed to assimilation in an attempt to escape reservation life.
1924	Citizenship and reorganization period. American Indians in 1924 became the last people given full citizenship and voting rights in the United States.
1934	The Indian Reorganization Bill gave American Indians the right to self-government but stipulated a discontinuation of land allotments; established provisions for education and training of American Indians.
1950–1960	Termination movement: an effort to end, tribe by tribe, any responsibility of the U.S. government for American Indian people, including health care. Accompanied by "relocation" of Indians from reservations to cities, where many became a part of the urban poor. Basically a new label for destruction of Indian communities and culture.
1955	American Indian health care is transferred to the Indian Health Service, a part of the Department of Health, Education, and Welfare.
1970	Indian Self-Determination Act. Allowed American Indian people to have more control over their governmental affairs.

(continued)

TABLE 2–1.	American Indians and Alaska Natives: significant dates and periods in recent history *(continued)*
Year(s)	**Periods and events**
1976	Indian Health Care Improvement Act. Intended to increase tribal input into health care; met with mixed results. It was administratively oriented and did not address topics such as traditional healing.
1980	The number of urban American Indian people surpasses the number of reservation and rural American Indian people.
1990	Staffing of the small Indian Health Service Mental Health program slated for increases. No specific programs for the elderly.

Source. Adapted from reference 6 and Baker FM, Lightfoot OB: "Psychiatric Care of Ethnic Elders," in *Culture, Ethnicity, and Mental Illness.* Edited by Gaw AC. Washington, DC, American Psychiatric Press, 1993.

American population was reduced to a mere 250,000 by 1850 (7).

- *Assimilation through the missionary system of education.* Both the sword and the cross were implemented by the European immigrants. Missionary schools were set up ostensibly to Christianize the Indian "heathens." In the enculturation process into Western culture, Indian children had to give up their languages, tribal customs and beliefs, and religion. The net result was a loss of continuity of native culture for generations of young Indians (7).

- *The forced boarding school experience.* Toward the end of the 1800s, Indian children were forcibly removed from their families to be "educated" at boarding schools. They were educated in Western culture, thoughts, and traditions. Native American parents and tribes were not given a voice in the matter of educating their children. The inadequate physical conditions of the schools, coupled with scarcity of food, lack of sanitation, overcrowding, and improper treatment of sick children, resulted in frequent epidemics. The experience not only produced several generations of Native Americans cut off from their family ties but also led to the development of "negative coping strategies" in order to survive. These strategies included learned helplessness, passive-aggressive behavior, manipulativeness, compulsive gambling, alcohol and drug abuse, suicide, denial, and scapegoating of other more successful Indians (7).

- *Urban relocation.* In the 1950s and 1960s, the federal government developed a termination/relocation plan that took many Indians from their homes and families and relocated them to various urban centers. Again, this forced method of assimilation led to cultural discontinuity and left a legacy of trauma experienced by Indians throughout the country (7).

These legacies left permanent scars in the psyche of the Native American people and serve as a backdrop for the psychological development of many Native Americans and their coping strategies in the mainstream of U.S. society.

■ DEMOGRAPHY

According to the U.S. Bureau of the Census, in 1990 there were 1.9 million American Indians, Eskimos, and Aleuts and 211,014 Native Hawaiians (8). These Native Americans belong to richly diverse subcultures based on tribal groups, geography, dialect, social patterns, and economic enterprise (8). More than 500 tribal groups, in 314 reservations with distinct languages, exist in the continental United States alone. About half of all Native Americans live on federal Indian reservations in 33 states; the other half live in urban areas. Children age 18 or younger compose about half of the Indian population. Most Hawaiian natives live on the islands of Hawaii. The states with largest number of American Indians are California, Oklahoma, New Mexico, Arizona, Alaska, North Carolina, and Washington. The Navajo reservation spans a large area that includes part of northern New Mexico and substantial areas of Arizona and Utah, for a total area far larger than the state of Connecticut. Other reservations, such as that of the Tewa tribe located within the city of El Paso, Texas, are quite small. Geographic diversity includes plains (South Dakota), northern woodlands (Manitoba, Canada), desert (New Mexico), and coastal areas (western coast of the northwestern United States, and British Columbia, Canada). Many tribes maintain their traditional languages, social and religious functions and ceremonies, family networks, close communion with nature, and traditional respect for children and elders.

In the United States, many Native American groups have sovereign nation status by virtue of the treaty between their tribes and the U.S. government. There is also a strong sentiment among Hawaiian natives to restore their sovereign nation status, a status that was lost when the Hawaiian monarchy was overthrown. Treaty obligations of the U.S. government include the provision of health services for Native Americans through the Indian Health Service (IHS). The IHS currently provides health services to approximately 60% of the Indian population (9). The federal budget allocated for mental health programs for Indians for fiscal year 1992 was $27.5 million. Since 1965, a system of ambulatory mental health services operated either by the IHS or by a tribe has gradually been developed (10). Most ambulatory services are crisis oriented and are provided by teams of mental health professionals with assistance from Native American mental health technicians who also serve as interpreters. Inpatient services, though limited, are usually provided under contract with local general hospitals or with private psychiatric hospitals. There is a great need for the provision of partial hospitalization, transitional living facilities, and child residential services (10). Because half of the Native American population consists of children, child specialists are in great demand to provide for their care.

Because North American Indians and Hawaiian natives have very different subcultures, I focus my discussion in this chapter only on cultural issues of those Native Americans residing in the continental United States.

■ NATIVE AMERICAN HEALTH BELIEFS AND CONCEPTION OF MENTAL ILLNESS

Walker and LaDue indicated that a "survival pact" is a set of guidelines for living that is a common thread among Indian people (6). The guidelines are based on the concept of a symbiosis, a coexistence and harmony between the individual, the group, and the earth, including all living things. The adherence to such a pact benefits all. Conversely, nonadherence puts all at risk and can result in the development of illnesses and calamities.

The conception of mental illness among Indian people varies with the degree of acculturation to the majority culture (5). Older Indians tend to adhere to traditional views, whereas younger Indians more often subscribe to Western beliefs.

As with humans from other backgrounds, Native Americans' conception of mental illness can be attributed to three causes: human, supernatural, and natural (11). Human causes include poisoning, wounds inflicted on self and others, and emotional losses. Supernatural causes include intrusion of spirits of animals, disrespect toward nature, ghosts, soul loss during dreams, omens, and taboos (11). Natural causes include accidents involving water, fire, and wind. The idea of unfulfilled dreams or desire, akin to the Western concept of unfulfilled unconscious libidinal drives, also has been mentioned (5).

■ DIAGNOSTIC ASSESSMENT INSTRUMENTS

Attempts have been made to assess the validity, compared with other cultures, of some standardized diagnostic instruments administered to Indian populations. Following are some of the findings:

1. *Thematic Apperception Test*. Results of Navajo males were compared with results from other cultures. Data showed comparable findings (12).
2. *Wechsler Intelligence Scale for Children, Revised*. Data showed some differences (13, 14).

3. *The Minnesota Multiphasic Personality Inventory.* Data showed limited usefulness in determining mental normalcy from mental illness and in distinguishing various types of mental illness (15).

4. *National Institute of Mental Health Center for Epidemiologic Studies Depression Scale.* May be a useful tool in targeting preventive intervention strategies with Indians, but its use as a screening instrument is suspect (16).

Limited, local, culturally relevant instruments that incorporate Indian cultural heritage and experiences also have been developed and found useful. One example is measures of life stress, locus of control, worldview, and values in Rosebud Sioux (17). Although some differences may be found in the interpretation of test results of standardized diagnostic instruments with Indians, many tests are still useful and their administration should be encouraged to assist diagnosis of mental illness, particularly when Indian cultural heritage and experience have been incorporated into the test (18).

■ EXPRESSION OF MENTAL ILLNESS

Epidemiological Data

There are no large-scale community survey data for the determination of prevalence and incidence of mental illness among Native Americans. Three small community epidemiological studies of Indians (from Saskatchewan, a U.S. Indian village, and an Eskimo community) were limited in scope, and therefore their findings cannot be generalized to most Indian communities (5). Depression, often complicated by the use of alcohol and other substances, seems to be the most common mental disorder in both adult and young Native Americans (10). There appears to be a high incidence of violent behaviors, including physical and sexual abuse of children, assault, homicide, and suicide in many Indian communities (10). The combination of low self-esteem, substance abuse, and frustration about living in an adverse environment have been contributory factors to these problems (10).

Studies show that Native Americans underutilize mental health services (19). In recent years, data on specific mental disorders in Indian tribes have appeared.

Affective Disorder

Shore and Manson (20) reported a high rate of depression among Native Americans. Furthermore, when a standard psychodiagnostic instrument was administered to a sample of individuals in three different tribal groups, Shore and colleagues (21) and Manson and colleagues (22) found a similar picture of depression across the three groups and found that the picture of depression is consistent with that in the majority cultures. The three major depression sub-groups identified were 1) an uncomplicated pattern, 2) secondary depression with a history of alcoholism, and 3) complicated depression superimposed on an underlying chronic depression or personality disorder (21, 22).

Indian suicide rates vary with age and gender. The Indian Health Service reported about 200 Indian suicides per year in 1989, with young males accounting for a large percentage of cases (23). Beiser and Attneave (24) also reported a high rate of suicides in Indian adolescents. When the pattern of health care utilization between Indians who completed suicide and those who attempted suicide were compared in a plains Indian reservation, those who completed suicide were less likely to have used clinical services provided by the IHS prior to death (25). The common methods used in completed suicide cases were firearms, hanging, and overdose (25). The need for programs to reach those at risk for completed suicide is evident.

Depression co-occurring with alcohol and marijuana use has been reported in a cohort of adolescents at a boarding school (26). Low suicide rates have been reported for older Indians, and suicide rates among Indian women were reported to be either low or comparable with those in the majority culture (5).

Alcohol and substance use and the presence of psychosis, depression, and social loneliness have been linked to Indian suicides.

Some of these suicides may be associated with single-car accidents and homicides (5).

Alcoholism and Substance Use

A high rate of alcoholism has been reported among Indian populations, particularly among males (24, 25). Prevalence rates of alcoholism vary by tribe and location as well as with the pattern of alcohol use (26, 27). For example, a higher alcoholism rate was found in the western part of Oklahoma than in the eastern part (5). Cases of alcoholism may be concentrated in pockets of population within a given community (5). About one-half of the adolescents detained in a juvenile detention center on a northern plains reservation had at least one alcohol, drug, or mental disorder diagnosis (28). In some tribes, severe alcohol use and its sequelae appear to start early in adolescence and tend to diminish with age (5). Alcoholism was found to have high comorbidity with cardiovascular diseases, hypertension, and diabetes in a Pacific Northwest Indian community (29). In a study (30) of the pattern of alcoholism in the Chippewa tribe as compared with the pattern among Caucasians, Westermeyer found that the Indian group showed more severe withdrawal phenomenon. This was attributed to possible delay in seeking treatment. As with cases of alcoholism in all populations, other factors such as a history of binge drinking, head trauma, intercurrent infection, and reduced access to treatment facilities as compared to access for Caucasians also have been implicated as contributing to the severe withdrawal phenomenon (5).

Despite extensive writings on the subject of the etiology of alcoholism in Indians, no convincing conclusions have been reached (5). However, the medical and social sequelae of alcoholism among Indian people are clear: alcoholism is seen as an important contributing factor for high rates of cirrhosis, automobile accidents, suicide, and homicide among Native Americans (5).

Other forms of substance use besides alcohol have been less studied. A survey of 35,000 Indian youths over age 12 revealed heavy use of marijuana, cocaine, phencyclidine (PCP), and other substances (31). Inhalant use among urban Native American youths in the Seattle metropolitan area was found to be less prevalent than use reported in most studies of youths at Indian reservations (32). As with other studies of inhalant abuse among youths, Native American youths who frequently used inhalants were associated with aggressivity, delinquency, sensation seeking, negative emotionality, conduct disorder, and alcohol dependence (32).

Psychosis

Psychosis among Indians is not well studied. The presence of auditory hallucinations per se may not be indicative of a mental disorder, particularly if it occurs within the context of an uncomplicated grief or a religious ritual. Although the content of delusions and hallucinations may be influenced by Indian culture, generally, the expression of psychoses among Indians is thought to be similar to the expression among those in the majority culture (5).

In a study (33) of 16 Indian patients in an IHS facility, males with diagnoses of schizophrenia presented with an increased potential for violence, and females frequently presented with withdrawn behavior. Kaplan and Johnson pointed out that clinicians should be alerted to the presence of extreme behaviors, such as those just mentioned, as heralding the need for treatment (34).

Disorders Usually First Evident in Childhood

Data on mental disorder among Indian children remain equivocal, with rates ranging from "low" to about one-third of Indian youth (5). Beiser and Attneave (35) found a higher risk for Indian children ages 5–9 entering the treatment system compared with Caucasian children. They also reported a high rate of suicide in Indian adolescents. In a 3-month prevalence study in southern Appalachia, Costello and colleagues (36) found higher rates of substance use and of comorbid substance use and psychiatric disorder among Indian youths compared with a sample of Caucasian youths. Data of Indian children with psychiatric disorders that relied on non-

Indian observer reports may be fraught with methodological problems. A recent study (37) compared depression and conduct disorder symptoms of North American native children in four different Indian settings across North America, with nonnative North American children, all in grades 2 and 4, as rated by teachers, parents, and self-reports of the children. The results revealed that the children rated themselves as having higher levels of depression than the adults rated them as having. Both the parents' reports and the children's self-reports revealed no differences in levels of conduct disorder symptoms between native and nonnative children. Nonnative teachers rated the native children as having higher levels of conduct disorder symptoms as compared with nonnative children. When the cultural distance between the observers and the subjects is taken into consideration, the study shows that there was possible observer bias when rating the native children. Furthermore, in a review of the psychiatric epidemiological literature on Indian children, Green and colleagues noted that some studies quoted figures for the prevalence of mental illness as ranging from "low" to one-third of Indian youth. These studies seldom used standard categories of psychopathology and instead relied on indices such as child abuse, delinquency, and school problems to reflect mental problems (38). The lack of correlations with fetal alcohol syndrome, substance use, depression, and the psychosocial condition of the mother (e.g., teenage pregnancy and teenage unemployment) further complicate analysis of true prevalence of mental illness among Indian children (5).

Culture-Bound Syndromes

Several culture-bound syndromes have been reported among Indians. The reader is referred to Chapter 4, Culture-Bound Syndromes, for a general discussion of the concept and various categories and to Simons and Hughes's classic description of culture-bound syndrome (39). Two of the better known culture-bound syndrome categories among Indians are *pibloktoq* and *windigo*.

Pibloktoq

Pibloktoq, also known as *Arctic hysteria,* affects women more than men. Found among the Arctic and Subarctic Eskimos, *pibloktoq* is characterized by abrupt episodes of extreme excitement, often followed by apparent seizures and transient coma. Prodromal symptoms of tiredness, depressive silences, vagueness of expression, and confusion for several days may precede attacks. During attacks, afflicted individuals may exhibit motor and verbal behavioral symptoms such as tearing off clothes and becoming partially or completely nude, supernatural strength, glossolalia, fleeing, rolling in snow, jumping into water, picking up and throwing things, performing mimetic acts and engaging in choreiform movements, and coprophagia. Following attacks, individuals may weep, manifest body tremor, become feverish, have a high pulse rate, and then sleep for many hours. Rational behavior resumes after rest (see also Chapter 4, Culture-Bound Syndromes).

Windigo

Windigo is a term that has been popularly associated with the idea of cannibal compulsion, an intense compulsive desire to eat human flesh, or one who develops craving for human flesh or is considered to be in the process of doing so (40). First introduced as a "sickness" by J. E. Saindon, an Oblate missionary who worked among the Cree of western James Bay in the early part of the twentieth century, the syndrome has been considered a cultural trait of the Northern Algonkian peoples for almost half a century. As an idiom of distress, *windigo* has been associated with "terrifying windstorms and uprooted trees and metaphorically extended to terrifying expression of uncontrolled human rage" (40, p. 414). The idea is "often related to the mystery and great concerns over a lost person" (40, p. 414). Because a person labeled *windigo* is considered to have broken a taboo against cannibalism, such an individual could be the projected object of group anxiety and therefore be killed or executed.

Morano recently reviewed 70 cases of "windigo psychosis" following 5 years of fieldwork among the Northern Ojibwa and the

Cree and could document only one case of murder-cannibalism under starvation conditions. His thesis is that the "*windigo* belief complex evolved among the Northern Algonkians as a way to help minimize the chances of getting caught in a famine with those who had already broken the taboo against cannibalism, to minimize the liabilities imposed by the incapacitated, and to focus group anxieties and aggressions upon individuals adjudged socially expendable" (40, p. 418).

At present, there is no conclusive evidence to consider *windigo* a culture-bound syndrome. It could be a variant of an obsessive-compulsive disorder. At best, it is an idiom of distress unique among the Algonkian people (see Chapter 4, Culture-Bound Syndromes, for the proposed criteria for these syndromes).

■ FAMILY RESPONSE TO MENTAL ILLNESS

To Native Americans, "family represents the cornerstone for the social and emotional well-being of individuals and communities" (41). Both parents are responsible for the care of their children and their aged parents, and close kinsmen are often relied upon to provide support. Extended family is typical of American Indians, and the grandparents often assume the roles of caregiver, trainer, and disciplinarian. Children often relate primarily to grandparents. Once married into a family, one is "blended" into the natural family, and not considered an "in-law" (41).

One difference from other North American families is that children are given relatively much more autonomy; sometimes this may appear uncaring and callous to non-Indian health workers (42). With more contact with Caucasians and health education, the pattern of Indian parents giving children autonomy may be changing.

Because of family orientation and emphasis on relationships, Indian families respond well to family and group therapeutic approaches, particularly when nondirective therapeutic approaches incorporate storytelling and metaphors (41).

In addition to family and informal tribal resources, Thompson and colleagues noted the involvement of multiple systems specifically designed for the care of Indian patients. The IHS, tribally run programs, and Western public and private medical and social service agencies are some examples (5).

■ TREATMENT OF AMERICAN INDIANS

Traditional Forms of Healing and Medicines

Certain myths and misconceptions have been perpetuated in the media regarding traditional Indian healers. It is widely recognized that the Indian medicine man or woman plays a key role in tribal life through the performance of healing ceremonies and worship and other roles such as priest, counselor, historian, and physician (5). Contrary to some popular myths and the writings of some anthropologists—and with few exceptions, such as some Mexican healers who may perform witchcraft against those who have broken social rules—most medicine men and women do not practice witchcraft, black magic, or sorcery (5). Their role centers primarily in healing and worship.

Indian medicines and traditional forms of healing existed long before European contact. Native people have long used herbal medicines for their laxative, emetic, diuretic, antipyretic, cardiac stimulant, and other medical effects (5).

Traditional healing practices take many forms and include sweats and other ceremonies and feasts. These ceremonies serve both preventive and curative purposes and provide group catharsis and relaxation for the benefits of both the individual and the group. Healing rituals include use of charms, amulets, and instruments with symbolic healing power accompanied by prayers, songs, and dances (5).

A *sweat,* used for prayer, cleansing, and healing, is held in a small space, such as a teepee. Steam is created in this space by pouring water over hot rocks (5). Feasts may be performed as a symbolic feeding to appease offended beings such as animals (5).

The *spirit dance* of the coast Salish and the *sun dance* of the Sioux focus on individual autonomy, strong kinship ties, community unification and affirmation of ancestral continuity, and guidelines and alternatives for behavior. The spirit dance requires abstinence from alcohol and drugs for an extended period of time and has been developed by native healers to address the problem of alcoholism (43).

There have been recent attempts to forge collaboration between practitioners of Western medicine and traditional Indian medicine. In a study of 60 cases of such collaboration, Manson noted some inherent difficulties from both sides of treatment. Problems defining what constitutes abnormality or legitimate traditional practice, explanatory models, credibility, reimbursements, the patient's expectations and consent, and professional biases all seem to hinder genuine collaboration. Such a model of collaboration cannot follow the usual way clinicians relate to other Western practitioners. Success will require careful arrangements of collaborative mechanisms in each local setting (5).

Cross-Cultural Psychopharmacological Issues of Native Americans

Some data are available concerning the genetic variations in enzymes involved in the metabolism of various psychotropic drugs among several native tribes in the United States (44). Individuals identified as having reduced metabolism of certain drugs (poor metabolizers) are at increased risk of developing potential side effects from dosages of psychotropic medications that are appropriate for individuals with normal amounts of metabolizing enzymes (extensive metabolizers) (see Chapter 6, Cross-Cultural Psychopharmacology). Table 2–2 shows the percentage of polymorphic poor metabolizing enzymes among certain Indian groups in North, Central, and South America (45, 46).

Because these enzymes (debrisoquine 4-hydroxylase, S-mephenytoin 4-hydroxylase, N-acetyltransferase, $ALDH_1$) are actively involved in the metabolism of most psychotropic drugs and their transport through serum (α-1-acid glycoprotein) (see Chapter 6, Cross-Cultural Psychopharmacology), the potential effects and side effects of their use in American Indians should be noted.

TABLE 2–2. **Percentage of poor metabolizing enzymes among American Indians**

American Indian group	Deb	Meph	N-Ace	ALDH$_1$	S-Var
North American Indians					
Eskimos	—	5–21	5–59	43–45	43
Canadian Indians	—	—	8	—	45
Navajo (New Mexico)	—	—	—	2	—
Sioux (North Dakota)	—	—	—	5	—
Oklahoma Indians	—	—	—	16	—
Central American Indians					
Mestizo (Mexico City)	—	—	—	4	54
Cuna (Panama)	0	0	24	—	—
Teribe (Panama)	—	—	29	—	—
Ngawbe Guaymi (Panama)	5.2	—	—	—	—
South American Indians					44
Atacamenos (Chile)	—	—	—	43	—
Mapuche (Chile)	—	—	—	41	—
Shuara (Ecuador)	—	—	22	42	—

Note. Deb = debrisoquine 4-hydroxylase deficiency; Meph = *S*-mephenytoin 4-hydroxylase deficiency; N-Ace = *N*-acetyltransferase; ALDH$_1$ = acetaldehyde dehydrogenase; S-Var = α-1-acid glycoprotein S variant.
Source. Adapted from references 45 and 46.

Treatment of Indian Patients by Non-Indian Therapists

Clinicians and researchers knowledgeable in the treatment of Indian patients have pointed out some of the inherent difficulties and pitfalls often encountered by non-Indian counselors:

- An unwitting assumption that the patient accepts all the values of the dominant culture (47)
- Patient underutilization of existing mental health services (19)
- Patient perception that existing services, where available, are not responsive
- Negative attitudes (fear, mistrust) of patients toward the presence of non-Indian counselors
- Patient unawareness of the kinds of counseling services available
- Preference of some patients for more traditional forms of healing

- Different beliefs and worldviews about the etiology of mental illness
- A lack of trained Indian, including Alaskan native, professionals in psychiatry, psychology, and social work; a heavy reliance on paraprofessional counselors in the IHS
- A paucity of research-oriented literature concerning the counseling process with Indians

Clevenger mentioned several aspects of the cultural experience of American Indians that are worth noting (42):

1. "The American Indian is a survivor of change" (42, p. 150). Indian tribes and culture have survived despite the encroachment on Indian reservations by Caucasians, conquest of Indian tribes by the U.S. military, relocation of Indian families to urban areas in the United States, "deculturation" of Indians by missionaries, and the raising of Indian children in boarding schools.
2. "The American Indian has a special sense of autonomy" (42, p. 151). Clevenger related an experience indicating an Indian's respect for the decision of her minor child; an Indian mother may consult her child about key medical decisions even though the child's response may be contradictory to the opinion of the professional, a behavior that can be foreign to a Western practitioner. In another case Clevenger related the experience of a psychiatrist questioning an Indian woman about her husband's reaction to his father's death. The woman answered, "I don't know—he didn't say." As an Indian, she would not presume to speak for her husband or anyone else. The information may have to be obtained and bereavement be interpreted through asking about collateral or circumstantial happenings related to her husband following the death of her father-in-law regarding changes in work habits, presence of depression, or a change of job and returning to the reservation (42, p. 151). Because Indian patients may not ask many questions, information and instructions about health procedures may have to be obtained and conveyed through significant others (42).

3. "The American Indian exists in a complex social structure" (42, p. 151). The clan to which an Indian belongs may be very extensive, with unique mythology, history, and political power.

4. "The American Indian has a complex spiritual reality" (42, p. 152). Art, music, and poetry as well as weaving, painting, and jewelry making are very much part of the Native American's daily life. So is a healing system that combines medicine with art and drama in ceremonies. Harmony with nature is emphasized and is conceptualized as a state of health. Disharmony with the universe may be perceived as cause for misfortune, accident, and illness (42).

5. "The American Indian has a long and unique history of dealing with the United States government" (42, p. 155). Through long experience with the former Bureau of Indian Affairs (and now with the IHS) and with the National Institute of Mental Health, American Indians have learned that the U.S. government's policies and procedures regarding them may not meet, or may be in conflict with, their needs. This can be reflected in a general mistrust of those in power. When working with native patients, as with all patients, trust must be earned and cultivated.

6. "Indians may have a different concept of time and ownership" (41). Because some Indians consider time to be "flowing" and "flexible," they may have difficulty adhering to the Western need for promptness in keeping appointments (5). Tardiness should not be automatically construed as a lack of care about their health problems or as "acting out" behavior in a psychodynamic sense. Also, during treatment, emphasis should be placed on present-day issues, rather than those in the future. The Indian concept of ownership is often focused on caretaking and sharing, not material goods. Schmidt cited this as a reason why Indians prefer to care for patients at home rather in a nursing home (5).

Tips for Non-Indian Therapists When Treating Native American Patients

The following are tips that non-Indian therapists can use when treating Native American patients:

1. When applying conventional psychotherapeutic technique to Indian patients, be mindful that the therapist will need to be sensitive and flexible and must incorporate the understanding of the ecology of Indian communities and the culture of origin an Indian brings to the counseling situation (48). Many Indians adhere to a holistic view of health and illness. It behooves therapists to explore etiological factors in the realm of the body, mind, and spirit. Scheduling of appointments should be made more flexible to accommodate the Indian sense of time. Focusing on present-day issues and fostering the development of problem-solving skills are good places to start.

2. Understanding the "cultural context" of the Indian patient's problem is a way to promote empathy in the counseling process. Familial patterns, peer-group orientations, socialization emphases, and tribal identifications provide some of the thread of this context (48). Group-oriented therapies are a culturally familiar technique of intervention. All tribes maintain a deep reverence for nature and a belief in a supreme force.

3. Seek consultation when needed. Consult formal and informal resources for mental health–related matters, particularly when complex problems arise. Formal resources such as the tribe and the IHS, as well as informal resources such as the family, traditional healers, and the shaman, can be called upon for assistance.

4. Consider possible assistance from traditional healers. Several authors emphasized the preference of some Indian patients to use some form of traditional healing approach when receiving treatment for emotional and behavioral problems (48).

5. Be familiar with some traditional tribal mannerisms and their role in communication. Clevenger mentioned the special sense of autonomy of American Indians. Direct eye contact may be a sign of disrespect for some Indians and may generate anxiety (42).

6. Clarify behavioral expectations for the patient in the counseling process. Trimble mentioned that some Indian patients simply do not know what is expected of them in the counseling situ-

ation. As with many ethnic patients, what constitutes expected patient behavior might need to be explicated. The relative "passivity" of some Indian patients is cited as an example of behavior that may require the therapist to be more creative in encouraging the patient to engage more actively in the counseling process. Is the individual problem reflective of a group problem? How should the group be engaged in providing venues for individual changes? These are issues to be explored (48).

7. Beware of countertransference. This could come in the form of biases about cultural pluralism that might interfere with the clinician-patient relationship (48). The therapist needs to examine his or her own worldview and values to recognize any potential conflict with those of the Indian patient.

8. Beware of potential variation in response to psychotropic drugs. As with other ethnic groups, variations in the pattern of responses to usual dosages of psychotropic drugs prescribed for the Caucasian population may exist owing to the existence of polymorphic metabolic enzymes. Such genetic variability may be reflected in either low or high serum drug levels, with consequential drug toxicity or lessened drug effects.

Implications for Training

In many training institutions, trainees barely have the opportunity to treat Native Americans and their families. Often, cases are haphazardly assigned. It is conceivable that a trainee may graduate from a program without ever treating a native person and his or her family.

Thompson has provided an outline for a cross-cultural curriculum for psychiatric residency programs that is appropriate for the treatment of Native Americans (49). Such a curriculum includes a more systematic way of assigning cases and training clinicians that encourages educational exposure to Native Americans and other minority patients. The following also would be required for a cross-cultural curriculum regarding Native Americans:

1. *Development and recruitment of cross-cultural faculties.* Many training institutions are located in inner cities where many urban Native Americans reside. It is important to first develop a faculty that includes members who are informed about the cultural issues of American Indian patients in their catchment area. A close interdisciplinary collaboration of psychiatrists, psychologists, social workers, psychiatric nurses, and anthropologists could provide cross-fertilization of knowledge and expertise. Interested faculty members should be involved in research activities that delineate cultural influence in psychiatric care. Teaching formats could include seminars, reading materials, research publications, case conferences, grand rounds topics, and guest speakers. The administration must actively support such ethnic-oriented programs and the care of patients from native and other ethnic backgrounds.

2. *More systematic assignment of native and ethnic patients and their families to residents, students, and other trainees so that trainees are exposed to as great a variety of patients from different backgrounds as possible.* Trainees should have the experience of engaging in psychotherapy with patients having a variety of ethnic backgrounds. In areas where there is a dearth of certain ethnic backgrounds, the existing cases could be shared among trainees through group discussion and supervision.

3. *Integration of cultural information.* Trainees should be encouraged to systematically incorporate ethnographic materials and community resources concerning the understanding and treatment of psychiatric problems of patients from native and other ethnic backgrounds. Anamnesis of cases and discussion should be expanded to include pertinent cultural factors such as those illustrated in this chapter. The use of the DSM-IV cultural formulation outline should be encouraged.

4. *Promotion of research.* Both faculty and trainees should be encouraged to conduct research and publish in the area of cross-cultural psychiatry, including psychiatric care of Native Americans.

■ CONCLUSION

Ethnic issues surrounding the psychiatric care of Native Americans has been selected as a paradigm to illustrate how cultural factors can be integrated into the psychiatric care of patients with ethnic varied backgrounds. Because of the lack of trained professionals available to treat Native American patients, there is an urgent need for more culturally competent mainstream clinicians to deliver care to native people and other minority groups. Developing cultural competency through understanding of the cultural factors in the psychiatric care of Native American patients is a necessary first step.

Non-Indian therapists treating American Indian patients need to discard stereotypes perpetuated by the media and a eurocentric historical perspective. The worldview of the native people and their historical encounters and experiences with nonnatives must be respected and understood. A nonjudgmental attitude and careful exploration of all aspects of Indian cultural life, including the gathering of information from different sources, goes a long way toward establishing trust and rapport with the American Indian patient. Clinical information should be augmented by readings about the respective Indian tribes. Consultation with therapists experienced in treating Indian patients and with traditional Indian healers is encouraged.

■ REFERENCES

1. Schermerhorn RA: Comparative Ethnic Relations: A Framework for Theory and Research. Chicago, IL, University of Chicago Press, 1970
2. Kleinman A: Rethinking Psychiatry. New York, Free Press, 1998
3. Gaw AC (ed): Culture, Ethnicity, and Mental Illness. Washington, DC, American Psychiatric Press, 1993

4. Harwood A (ed): Ethnicity and Medical Care. Cambridge, MA, Harvard University Press, 1981

5. Thompson JW, Walker DR, Silk-Walker P: Psychiatric care of American Indians and Alaska Natives, in Culture, Ethnicity, and Mental Illness. Edited by Gaw AC. Washington, DC, American Psychiatric Press, 1993, pp 189–243

6. Walker RD, LaDue R: An integrative approach to American Indian mental health, in Ethnic Psychiatry. Edited by Wilkinson CB. New York, Plenum, 1986

7. Tafoya N, Del Vecchio A: Back to the future: an examination of the Native American holocaust experience, in Ethnicity and Family Therapy, 2nd Edition. Edited by McGoldrick M, Giordano J, Pearce JK. New York, Guilford Press, 1996, pp 45–55

8. U.S. Bureau of the Census: 1990 Census Profile: Race and Hispanic Origin. Washington, DC, Population Division, U.S. Bureau of the Census.

9. Johnson KW, Anderson NB, Bastida E, Kramer BJ, Williams D, Wong M: Panel II: macrosocial and environmental influences on minority health. Health Psychol 14:601–612, 1995

10. Nelson SH, McCoy GF, Stetter M, Vanderwagen WC: An overview of mental health services for American Indians and Alaska Natives in the 1990s. Hospital and Community Psychiatry 43:257–261, 1992

11. Vogel VJ: American Indian Medicine. Norman, OK, University of Oklahoma Press, 1970

12. Goldstine T, Gutmann D: A TAT study of Navajo aging. Psychiatry 35:373–384, 1972

13. Browne DB: WISC-R scoring patterns among Native Americans of the northern plains. White Cloud Journal 3:3–16, 1984

14. McShane DA, Plas JM: WISC-R factor structures for Ojibwa Indian children. White Cloud Journal 2:18–22, 1982

15. Pollack D, Shore JH: Validity of the MMPI with Native Americans. Am J Psychiatry 137:946–950, 1980

16. Baron AE, Manson SM, Ackerson LM, et al: Depressive symptomatology in older American Indians with chronic disease:

some psychometric considerations, in Depression in Primary Care: Screening and Detection. Edited by Atkinsson C, Zich JM. New York, Routledge, 1990, pp 217–231

17. Dana RH, Hornby R, Hoffmann T: Local norms of personality assessment for Rosebud Sioux. White Cloud Journal 3:17–25, 1984

18. Manson SM, Walker RD, Kivlahan DR: Psychiatric assessment and treatment of American Indians and Alaska Natives. Hospital and Community Psychiatry 38:165–173, 1987

19. Sue S: Community mental health services to minority groups: some optimism, some pessimism. Am Psychol 32:616–624, 1977

20. Shore JH, Manson SM: Cross-cultural studies of depression among American Indians and Alaska Natives. White Cloud Journal 2:5–12, 1981

21. Shore JH, Manson SM, Bloom JD, et al: A pilot study of depression among American Indian patients with research diagnostic criteria. Am Indian Alsk Native Ment Health Res 1:4–15, 1987

22. Manson SM, Shore JH, Bloom JD: The depressive experience in American Indian communities: a challenge for psychiatric theory and diagnosis, in Culture and Depression. Edited by Kleinman A, Good B. Berkeley, CA, University of California Press, 1985

23. Indian Health Service: Trends in Indian Health, 1989. Rockville, MD, U.S. Department of Health and Human Services, Program Statistics Branch, Indian Health Service, 1989

24. Beiser M, Attneave CL: Mental disorders among Native American children: rates and risk periods for entering treatment. Am J Psychiatry 139(2):193–198, 1982

25. Dinges NG, Duong-Tran Q: Stressful life events and co-occurring depression, substance abuse and suicidality among American Indian and Alaska Native adolescents. Cult Med Psychiatry 16:487–502, 1992 93

26. Stratton R, Zeiner A, Paredes A: Tribal affiliation and prevalence of alcohol problems. J Stud Alcohol 39:1167–1177, 1978

27. Westermeyer J: "The drunken Indian": myths and realities. Psychiatric Annals 4:29–36, 1974
28. Duclos CW, Beals J, Novins DK, et al: Prevalence of common psychiatric disorders among American Indian adolescent detainees. J Am Acad Child Adolesc Psychiatry 37:866–873, 1998
29. Boehnlein JK, Kinzie DJ, Leong PK, et al: The natural history of medical and psychiatric disorders in an American Indian community. Cult Med Psychiatry 16:543–554, 1992–93
30. Westermeyer J: Chippewa and majority alcoholism in the Twin Cities: a comparison. J Nerv Ment Dis 155:322–327, 1972
31. Beauvais F, Oetting ER, Edwards RW: Trends in drug use of Indian adolescents living on reservations: 1975–1983. Am J Drug Alcohol Abuse 11:209–230, 1985
32. Howard MO, Walker DR, Walker PS, et al: Inhalant use among urban American Indian youth. Addiction 94:83–95, 1999
33. Levy J: Quoted in Kunitz SJ: Disease Change and the Role of Medicine: The Navajo Experience. Berkeley, CA, University of California Press, 1983
34. Kaplan B, Johnson D: The social meaning of Navajo psychopathology, in Magic, Faith, and Healing. Edited by Kiev A. New York, Free Press, 1964
35. Beiser M, Attneave CL: Mental disorders among Native American children: rates and risk periods for entering treatment. Am J Psychiatry 139:193–198, 1982
36. Costello JE, Farmer EMZ, Angold A, et al: Psychiatric disorders among American Indian and white youth in Appalachia: the Great Smokey Mountains Study. Am J Public Health 87:827–832, 1997
37. Dion R, Gotowiec A, Beiser M: Depression and conduct disorder in native and non-native children. J Am Acad Child Adolesc Psychiatry 37:736–742, 1998
38. Green BE, Sack WH, Pambrun A: A review of child psychiatric epidemiology with special reference to American Indian and Alaska Native children. White Cloud Journal 2:22–36, 1981
39. Simons RC, Hughes CC (eds): The Culture-Bound Syndrome. Dordrecht, Holland, D. Reidel, 1985

40. Marano L: *Windigo* psychosis: the anatomy of an emic-etic confusion, in The Culture-Bound Syndrome. Edited by Simons RC, Hughes CC. Dordrecht, Holland, D. Reidel, 1985, pp 411–448

41. Sutton CT, Broken Nose MA: American Indian Families: an overview, in Ethnicity and Family Therapy, 2nd Edition. Edited by McGoldrick M, Giordano J, Pearce JK. New York, Guilford Press, 1996, pp 31–44

42. Clevenger J: Native Americans, in Cross-Cultural Psychiatry. Edited by Gaw A. Boston, John Wright-PSG, 1982, pp 149–161

43. Walker DR, Lambert DM, Walker PS, Kivlahan DR: Treatment implications of comorbid psychopathology in American Indians and Alaska Natives. Cult Med Psychiatry 16:555–572, 1993

44. Mendoza R, Smith MW, Poland RE, et al: Ethnic psychopharmacology: the Hispanic and Native American perspective. Psychopharmacol Bull 27:449–461, 1991

45. Agarwal DP, Goedde HW: Alcohol Metabolism, Alcohol Intolerance, and Alcoholism. Berlin, Springer-Verlag, 1990

46. Eap CB, Bauman P: The genetic polymorphism of human alpha-1-acid glycoprotein: genetics, biochemistry, physiological functions, and pharmacology. Prog Clin Biol Res 300:111–125, 1989

47. Bryde JF: Indian Students and Guidance. Boston, Houghton-Mifflin, 1971

48. Trimble JE, Lafrombois T: American Indians and the counseling process: culture, adaptation, and style, in Handbook of Cross-Cultural Counseling and Therapy. Edited by Pedersen P. Greenwood Press, Westport, CT, 1985

49. Thompson JW: A curriculum for learning about American Indians and Alaska natives in psychiatry residency training. Academic Psychiatry 20:5–12, 1996

3

CULTURE IN DSM-IV

Cultural issues are considered for inclusion in DSM-IV (1) in five different domains. Mezzich et al. (2) outlined the major cultural contributions to DSM-IV as follows:

1. Cultural statement for the introduction to the manual
2. Cultural considerations for various diagnostic categories
3. Cultural annotations for the multiaxial schema
4. Cultural formulation guidelines
5. Glossary of culture-bound syndromes and idioms of distress

In this chapter I summarize the specific cultural contribution in each of the diagnostic categories of DSM-IV. Additionally, I discuss the significance of the cultural statement in the introduction to the manual and the cultural annotations of the multiaxial schema. Other cultural contributions are discussed in separate chapters in this book: Chapter 4, Culture-Bound Syndromes, and Chapter 5, Cultural Formulation.

One of the important contributions of DSM-IV is the requirement for the clinician to take into consideration cultural context when making a diagnosis. Thus, information on cultural variations in distress idioms, symptom patterns, dysfunctions, correlates, and course of the disorder must be taken into account to ascertain whether the diagnostic criteria are applicable to the patient (2).

The following is a summary of the specific cultural considerations in DSM-IV diagnostic catagories. In DSM-IV each diagnostic category is included under a section heading "Specific Culture, Age, and Gender Features." In this chapter only the cultural information of each diagnostic category that is available in DSM-IV is summarized. Age and gender information is omitted. Where no cultural information is provided in the diagnostic category, that category is excluded from this chapter.

■ SPECIFIC CULTURAL CONSIDERATIONS IN DSM-IV DIAGNOSTIC CATEGORIES

The following is a summary of the key cultural features in each diagnostic category of DSM-IV.

Disorders Usually First Diagnosed in Infancy, Childhood, or Adolescence

Mental Retardation and Learning Disorders

Because individualized testing is always required to make the diagnosis of mental retardation or learning disorder, care should be taken to ensure that intelligence testing procedures have been validated across cultural groups. The individual's relevant ethnic and cultural characteristics should be represented in the standardization sample of the tests. Examiners who are familiar with aspects of the individual's ethnic or cultural background should be employed to perform the testing.

*Language Disorder and Phonological Disorder
(Formerly Developmental Articulation Disorder)*

Care must be exercised when making judgments about expressive language disorders of individuals growing up in a non-English speaking or bilingual environment. The standardized measures of language development and of nonverbal intellectual capacity must be relevant for the patient's cultural and linguistic group. The examiner should be familiar with the patient's cultural and linguistic contexts in the assessment of the development of communication abilities.

Conduct Disorder

Misapplication of the conduct disorder diagnosis to individuals in settings in which patterns of undesirable behavior are sometimes viewed as protective—as in high-crime, impoverished areas—should be avoided. It is important to distinguish whether a behavior is symptomatic of an underlying dysfunction or simply a reaction to a difficult environment.

Pica

In some cultures, the eating of dirt or other seemingly nonnutritive substances is believed to be of value.

Tourette's Disorder

Tourette's disorder has been widely reported as occurring in diverse racial and ethnic groups.

Separation Anxiety Disorder

The degree to which it is considered desirable to tolerate separation varies across cultures. In some cultures, interdependence among rather than independence from family members is highly valued.

Selective Mutism

Care should be exercised not to misdiagnose immigrant children with selective mutism when they are unfamiliar with or uncomfortable with the official language of their new host country and refuse to speak to strangers in their new environment.

Delirium, Dementia, and Amnestic and Other Cognitive Disorders

Delirium

The evaluation of an individual's mental capacity should include his or her cultural and educational background. Individuals from diverse cultural backgrounds may not be familiar with the information normally used in a mental status examination. Certain tests of general knowledge (e.g., names of presidents, geographic location), abstraction (e.g., proverbs), memory (e.g., date of birth, because some cultures do not celebrate birthdays), and orientation (e.g., sense of placement, because location may be conceptualized differently) are useless if the information being requested is unfamiliar to the individual.

Dementia

Unfamiliarity with the test items mentioned above also applies to the diagnosis of dementia because of the variations in cultural and educational background of certain individuals. In addition, the prevalence of different causes of dementia (e.g., infections, nutritional deficiencies, traumatic brain injury, endocrine disturbances, cerebrovascular diseases, seizure disorders, brain tumors, substance abuse) varies considerably across cultural groups.

Mental Disorders Due to a General Medical Condition

Substance Intoxication

Wide cultural variation exists in attitudes toward drug use, in patterns of substance use, in accessibility of substances, in physiological reactions to substances, and in the prevalence of substance-related disorders. The acceptance of mood-altering drugs varies across different ethnic groups. Exposure to substances and patterns of medication use also vary widely within and between countries.

Alcohol-Related Disorders

In different cultures, marked differences exist in the quantity, frequency, and pattern of alcohol consumption. Genetic differences may influence the prevalence of alcoholism. In most Asian cultures, the overall prevalence of alcohol-related disorders may be relatively low and the male-to-female ratio high. About 50% of Japanese, Chinese, and Korean individuals are deficient in the form of aldehyde dehydrogenase that eliminates low levels of the first breakdown product of alcohol, acetaldehyde. When such individuals consume alcohol, they experience a flushed face, palpitations, and dysphoria that discourages them from consuming large amounts of alcohol. In the United States, whites and African Americans have nearly identical rates of alcohol abuse and dependence. Latino males have somewhat higher rates, although prevalence is lower among Latino females than among females from other ethnic groups.

Amphetamine-Related Disorder Not Otherwise Specified

All levels of society show amphetamine dependence and abuse. This disorder is more common among persons between 18 and 30 years of age.

Caffeine-Induced Disorders

The pattern of caffeine use and the sources from which caffeine is obtained vary widely among different cultures. The average caffeine intake in most of the developing world is less than 50 mg/day, compared with as much as 400 mg/day or more in Sweden, the United Kingdom, and other European nations. Caffeine consumption increases during the 20s and often decreases after age 65. Intake is greater for males than for females.

Cannabis-Related Disorders

Considered probably the world's most commonly used illicit substance, cannabis has been taken since ancient times for its psychoactive effects and as a remedy for a wide range of medical conditions. Cannabis is among the first drugs of experimentation—a "gateway drug" (often in the teens)—for all cultural groups in the United States.

Cocaine-Related Disorders

All racial, socioeconomic, age, and gender groups in the United States are affected by cocaine use and its attendant disorders.

Hallucinogen-Related Disorders

Hallucinogens may be used as part of established religious rituals. There are regional differences in their use in the United States.

Opioid-Related Disorders

In the late 1800s and early 1900s, opioid dependence was seen more often among white middle-class individuals, suggesting that differences in use reflect the availability of opioid drugs and other social factors. Since the 1920s in the United States, there has been an overrepresentation of opioid dependence among members of minority groups living in economically deprived areas.

Phencyclidine-Related Disorders

Minority groups in the United States appear to have a twofold higher prevalence of phencyclidine-related problems.

Schizophrenia and Other Psychotic Disorders

Schizophrenia

The symptoms of schizophrenia, regarding content, course, and outcome, may vary across cultural groups. Care must be exercised in the determination of abnormality of experiences. Visual or auditory hallucinations with a religious content as part of a religious experience (e.g., seeing the Virgin Mary or hearing the voice of God) may not be delusional. Catatonic behavior appears to be more common in non-Western cultures compared with behaviors reported among individuals in the United States diagnosed as having schizophrenia. An acute course and a better outcome have been noted in individuals with schizophrenia in developing countries than in individuals in industrialized nations. This may result in higher rates of schizophreniform disorder than of schizophrenia. When assessing symptoms of schizophrenia, variation in linguistic style and presentation that influence speech, affect, and volition should be carefully considered so that bipolar disorders are not misdiagnosed as schizophrenia, as has been reported in some ethnic groups in the United States.

Delusional Disorder

The content of delusions varies in different cultures and subcultures. In the assessment of delusions, care must be taken in evaluating an individual's cultural and religious background. Some groups have widely and culturally sanctioned beliefs that might be considered delusional in other cultures.

Mood Disorders

The experience, expression, and communication of symptoms of depression and hypomania may vary across cultural groups. In some cultures, depression may be experienced largely in somatic terms, rather than in sadness or guilt. Depressive experiences may be expressed as complaints of weakness, tiredness, "imbalance" (in Chinese and Asian cultures), "nerves" and headaches (in Latino and Mediterranean cultures), or being "heartbroken" (among Hopi Native Americans). Judgment about the seriousness of the experience or expression of dysphoria may vary in different cultures. In some cultures, irritability may provoke greater concern than sadness or withdrawal. Culturally distinctive experiences (e.g., fear of being hexed or bewitched, feeling of "heat in the head" or crawling sensations of worms or ants, or being visited by deceased individuals) must be distinguished from actual hallucinations or delusions that may be part of symptoms of a major depressive episode, with psychotic disorder. Care should also be exercised not to simply dismiss a symptom merely because it is viewed as the "norm" for a culture. There are reports that some clinicians may have a tendency to underdiagnose bipolar disorder (and instead, diagnose it schizophrenia) in some ethnic groups in the United States.

Anxiety Disorders

Panic Disorder With or Without History of Agoraphobia

In certain cultures, panic attacks may be precipitated by intense fear of witchcraft or magic. In DSM-IV, some culture-bound syndromes such as *koro* may exhibit features of panic attack associated with fear of shrinkage of genitalia into the body (see Chapter 4, Culture-Bound Syndromes). In some cultures, women are restricted from participation in public life. This should not be confused with agoraphobia.

Specific Phobia

The content of phobias and their prevalence vary across cultures. In a culture that believes in magic, a specific phobia should be diagnosed only if the fear is excessive in the context of that culture and causes significant impairment or distress.

Social Phobia

The presentation of social phobia may vary across cultures. In some Asian cultures (Japan and Korea), instead of a marked persistent fear of social or performance situations in which embarrassment may occur (criterion A in DSM-IV-TR), some individuals may develop a persistent and excessive fear of giving offense to others in social situations. Such fears may take the form of extreme anxiety that blushing, eye-to-eye contact, or one's body odor will be offensive to others (a culture-bound syndrome called *taijin kyofusho,* in Japan) (see description in Chapter 4, Culture-Bound Syndromes).

Obsessive-Compulsive Disorder

Culturally prescribed ritual behavior should be distinguished from abnormal behavioral patterns of obsessive-compulsive disorder. Ritualistic behaviors of obsessive-compulsive disorder exceed cultural norms, occur at times and places judged inappropriate by others of the same culture, and interfere with social role functioning. Individuals may complain of the disruptive nature of these behaviors in their daily routines. Intensification of normative ritual behavior may occur during periods of mourning and important life transitions. These may appear as obsession to clinicians unfamiliar with the cultural context.

Posttraumatic Stress Disorder

Special care is needed in the assessment of immigrants from areas where the population is at high risk for posttraumatic stress disorder. Higher rates of posttraumatic stress disorder may be found in recent immigrants from areas with considerable social unrest and war. Further, these immigrants may be reluctant to divulge experiences of torture and trauma for fear of political repercussions or the risk of losing immigration status.

In younger children, the pattern of expressing traumatic experiences may be different from that of adults. Distressing dreams of the event may change into generalized nightmares of rescuing others or of threats to self or others. Reliving of the trauma may occur through repetitive play. There may be diminished interest in daily activities, constriction of affect, a sense of foreshortened future, a belief in an ability to foresee future untoward events (omen formation), or complaints of various physical symptoms such as stomachaches and headaches. Clinicians may have to rely on reports from parents, teachers, and other observers in the evaluation of these symptoms.

Acute Distress Disorder

Coping patterns for stress vary across cultures. In certain cultures, dissociative symptoms may be a more prominent part of the acute stress response if such behaviors are culturally sanctioned (e.g., *ataques de nervios* among Latinos, *amok* among Malays).

Generalized Anxiety Disorder

There are considerable cultural variations in the expression of anxiety. In some cultures, anxiety is expressed predominantly through somatic symptoms, whereas in others it is expressed through cognitive symptoms. The cultural context of the experience of anxiety should be taken into consideration when evaluating whether worries about certain situations are excessive.

Somatoform Disorders

Somatization Disorder

Manifestation of somatic symptoms may vary in content and frequency across cultures. In Africa and North Asia, more than in North America, the nondelusional experience of worms in the head or ants crawling under the skin has been reported. A culture-bound syndrome called *dhat* syndrome exists in India that reflects cultural concern about semen loss. Somatization disorder appears to occur in higher frequency among Puerto Rican and Greek men and only rarely among men in the United States.

Undifferentiated Somatoform Disorder

Personal and social problems often are expressed as idioms of distress in different cultures. However, these idioms do not necessarily indicate psychopathology. Variations in the presentation of certain medically unexplained symptoms characterized by fatigue and weakness for 6 months or longer is a frequent complaint in many parts of the world. Although classified as undifferentiated somatoform disorder in DSM-IV, clinicians in other nations frequently label this as *neurasthenia.*

Conversion Reaction

Conversion disorder is reported to be more common among individuals from rural areas, among those with lower socioeconomic status, and in individuals less knowledgeable about medical and psychological concepts. In addition, in certain cultures, falling down with loss or alteration of consciousness is an acceptable idiom of distress that is associated with a variety of culture-specific syndromes (see Chapter 4, Culture-Bound Syndromes). In certain culturally sanctioned religious and healing rituals, behavioral changes resembling conversion and dissociation are common. Clinicians should take the social context into consideration when judging the abnormality of these symptoms.

Pain Disorder

There is considerable variation among ethnic and cultural groups in their reaction to painful stimuli and in the way they express their reaction to pain. For example, in one classic study (3), compared with Irish patients, Italian patients presented with significantly more pain symptoms, had symptoms in significantly more bodily locations, and noted significantly more types of bodily dysfunctions.

Hypochondriasis

In certain cultures, hypochondriasis may persist because an individual's ideas about his or her disease may be reinforced by traditional healers who may disagree with the reassurance given by medical practitioners. Clinicians evaluating the unreasonableness for the preoccupation with the disease should take this into consideration.

Body Dysmorphic Disorder

Preoccupations about an imagined physical defect may be influenced or amplified by cultural factors. *Koro,* a culture-bound syndrome, has been reported primarily in Southeast Asia and is characterized by the preoccupation that the penis (or female genitalia) is shrinking and will disappear into the abdomen, resulting in death. *Koro* may be related to body dysmorphic disorder but differs from it by its usually brief duration, different associated symptom of panic and fear of death, positive response to reassurance, and occasional occurrence as an epidemic (see also *koro* in Chapter 4, Culture-Bound Syndromes).

Dissociative Disorders

Dissociative Fugue

Culture-bound syndromes characterized by *running syndromes* have been reported and are described as *pibloktoq* among arctic native people, *grisi siknis* among the Miskito of Honduras and Nicaragua, *frenzy* witchcraft among Navajo, and some form of *amok* in western Pacific cultures. These syndromes may meet criteria for dissociative fugue and are characterized by a sudden onset of a high level of activity, a trancelike state, potentially dangerous behavior in the form of running or fleeing (homicide in *amok*), and ensuing exhaustion, sleep, and amnesia for the episode (see Chapter 4, Culture-Bound Syndromes).

Dissociative Identity Disorder

The recent relatively high rates of dissociative identity disorder reported in the United States might suggest that this is a culture-bound syndrome.

Depersonalization Disorder

Clinicians should differentiate a culturally sanctioned, normative, voluntarily induced experience of depersonalization or derealization in meditative or trance practice from depersonalization disorder.

Dissociative Disorder Not Otherwise Specified

Possession identity disorder—which involves replacement of the customary sense of personal identity by a new identity attributed to the influence of a spirit, power, deity, another person, animal, or even inanimate object—has been reported in many cultures. Possession trance with stereotyped "involuntary" movements or amnesia may be associated with *amok* (Indonesia), *bebainan* (Indonesia), *latah* (Malaysia), *pibloktoq* (Arctic), *atague de nervios* (Latin America), and possession (India). Dissociative trance disorder should not be confused with normative-induced trance phenomena in cultural or religious practice.

Sexual and Gender Identity Disorders

Care should be taken in judging sexual dysfunction. An individual's ethnic, cultural, social, and religious background may influence sexual desire, expectations, and attitudes about performance. In some cultures, a higher premium is placed on fertility, and sexual desires on the part of women are given less relevance.

Paraphilia

Behavioral deviancy in one cultural setting may be more acceptable in another setting. This may complicate the diagnosis of paraphilia across cultural or religious groups.

Gender Identity Disorder

Societal responses to gender identity disorders within a specific culture may vary. Females with this disorder generally experience less ostracism because of cross-gender interests. They suffer less from peer rejection, at least until adolescence.

Eating Disorders

Anorexia Nervosa

Abundance of food and the cultural idea of attractiveness linked to thinness for females have been suggested for the higher prevalence of anorexia nervosa in industrialized societies. Immigrants who have assimilated the thin-body idea may likewise be affected. Cultural expression of the motivation for food restriction may vary: instead of a disturbed perception of the body, individuals may complain of epigastric discomfort or distaste for food.

Bulimia Nervosa

Most studies of bulimia nervosa have been done in industrialized countries. The prevalence of this disorder appears similar in most industrialized countries, including the United States, Canada, Europe, Australia, Japan, New Zealand, and South Africa.

Sleep Disorders

Nightmare Disorder

Interpretation of the significance of nightmares varies across cultures. Some cultures consider nightmares to be signs of spiritual or supernatural phenomena; others may relate it to mental or physical disturbance. A diagnosis of nightmare disorder should not be made unless there is persistent distress or impairment that warrants independent clinical attention.

Sleep Terror Disorder, Sleepwalking Disorder

Although the significance and cause of sleep terror disorder and sleepwalking disorder are thought to differ across cultures, no clear evidence currently exists.

Insomnia Related to Another Mental Disorder, Hypersomnia Related to Another Mental Disorder

Complaints of insomnia and hypersomnia may vary in different cultural groups depending on the degree of stigmatization of sleep complaint.

Impulse-Control Disorders Not Elsewhere Classified

Intermittent Explosive Disorder

Although *amok* as a culture-bound syndrome was first reported in Southeast Asia, isolated cases of *amok* have been reported in Canada and the United States. *Amok* typically is characterized as follows: Following a prodromal brooding period, a sudden outburst of unrestrained violent behavior occurs, which may result in homicides. The individual eventually becomes exhausted and claims amnesia afterward (see also *amok* in Chapter 4, Culture-Bound Syndromes).

Pathological Gambling

Different cultures have different types of gambling activities (e.g., cockfights, paigo, horse racing, stock market). Clinicians should tailor their treatment to fit the attitude toward gambling in the patient's cultural background and the particular activity gambled on.

Adjustment Disorders

Clinicians should consider an individual's cultural setting before making a diagnosis of adjustment disorder. The threshold for maladaptiveness varies because various cultures have different ways of experiencing and coping with stressors and interpreting the meanings of stressors.

Personality Disorders

Care should be exercised in diagnosing personality disorder in individuals from different cultural groups. In immigrants, the factors of acculturation and the individual's customary expression of habits, customs, or political or religious values from the culture of origin should be taken into consideration when determining deviancy. Individuals familiar with the person's cultural background may assist in providing additional information.

Paranoid Personality Disorder

Care should be exercised in diagnosing an individual as "paranoid," particularly for members of minorities, immigrants, political and economic refugees, and individuals from different ethnic backgrounds who display a guarded attitude or defensive behavior due to unfamiliarity with the culture of the host society or in response to perceived neglect or indifference. Clinicians may be perceived as "agents" of the host society, thus confounding the issue of mutual trust. These factors should be distinguished from true paranoid personality disorder.

Schizoid Personality Disorder

Inhibited or defensive behavior, as found in some immigrants or migrants, should not be labeled as schizoid. The phenomenon of *emotional freezing,* as an adjustment reaction to a new environment has been described in individuals moving from rural to metropolitan areas. This is characterized by solitary activities, constricted affect, and other deficits in communication and should be distinguished from schizoid personality disorder.

Schizotypal Personality Disorder

According to DSM-IV-TR, "the essential feature of schizotypal personality disorder is a pervasive pattern of social and interpersonal deficits marked by acute discomfort with, and reduced capacity for, close relationships as well as by cognitive or perceptual distortions and eccentricities of behavior" (1, p. 697). Care should be taken when these criteria are applied cross-culturally in the evaluation of cognitive and perceptual distortions. Pervasive culturally determined characteristics, particularly those relating to religious beliefs and rituals (e.g., voodoo, speaking in tongues, life beyond death, shamanism, mind reading, sixth sense, evil eye, magical beliefs related to health and illness) must be taken into consideration to avoid misdiagnosis.

Antisocial Personality Disorder

The social and economic context should be considered in assessing antisocial behaviors. In an urban setting, particularly among low socioeconomic groups, seemingly antisocial behavior may be part of a protective survival strategy. Clinicians should not misapply the antisocial personality disorder diagnosis to such individuals.

Borderline Personality Disorder

The pattern of behavior described in borderline personality disorder has been reported in many cultures.

Histrionic Personality Disorder

According to DSM-IV-TR, "the essential feature of histrionic personality disorder is pervasive and excessive emotionality and attention-seeking behavior" (1, p. 711). Norms for interpersonal behavior, personal appearance, and emotional expressiveness vary across cultures, gender, and age groups. It is important to take these into consideration when diagnosing histrionic personality disorder (1, p. 712).

Avoidant Personality Disorder

Caution should be exercised when diagnosing avoidant behavior. Different cultural and ethnic groups vary in the degree to which they regard diffidence and avoidance as appropriate. Immigrants may manifest avoidance behavior following immigration.

Dependent Personality Disorder

The degree of appropriateness of dependent behavior varies across age and cultural groups. Some cultures emphasize passivity, politeness, and deferential treatment. The cultural norm of the individual should be taken into consideration in determining whether dependent behavior is excessive.

Obsessive-Compulsive Personality Disorder

Culturally sanctioned habits, rituals, customs, work habits, or interpersonal styles should not be considered abnormal when assessing an individual for obsessive-compulsive personality disorder.

■ CULTURAL STATEMENT IN THE INTRODUCTION TO DSM-IV

A section titled "Ethnic and Cultural Considerations" is included in the introduction to DSM-IV. This section cautions clinicians to exercise sensitivity and to consider variations in behavior, belief, or experience when DSM-IV diagnostic categories are applied to individuals from a different ethnic or cultural group. Some culturally sanctioned experiences, such as hearing or seeing a deceased relative during bereavement, or auditory or visual hallucination in certain religious rituals, may be diagnosed as manifestations of a psychotic disorder if the clinician does not take the cultural context of the experience into consideration. Likewise, certain cultural groups may have a preferred idiom for expressing distress. Clinicians unfamiliar with these notions and idioms of distress may be at a loss for comprehending the nature of the complaints. Not only may there be a misdiagnosis, but culturally appropriate treatment modalities may be missed. Thus, it is essential to be familiar with an individual's cultural frame of reference when judging psychopathology.

The ethnic and cultural considerations section mentions inclusion of three types of information specifically related to cultural considerations in DSM-IV:

- A discussion in the text of cultural variations in each diagnostic category that has such information
- A glossary of the best-studied culture-bound syndromes
- An outline for cultural formulation

These efforts are intended to enhance cultural awareness and sensitivity in the use of DSM-IV in culturally diverse populations in the United States and in the world.

■ CULTURAL ANNOTATIONS IN MULTIAXIAL ASSESSMENT

Multiaxial assessment allows for the codification of a comprehensive assessment of the health and illness status of an individual. Rather than the traditional monolithic categorical classification of disease, DSM-IV adopts a five-axis assessment scheme. Each axis portrays a different domain of information:

Axis I:	Clinical disorders
	Other conditions that may be a focus of clinical attention
Axis II:	Personality disorders
	Mental retardation
Axis III:	General medical conditions
Axis IV:	Psychosocial and environmental problems
Axis V:	Global assessment of functioning

Clinicians are encouraged to consider cultural factors in the assessment of each axis (2). Examples of the cultural variation in the presentation of Axes I and II categories have been already addressed in this chapter. Cultural and ethnic variation involving genetic factors in sickle anemia among African Americans and Africans (2), glucose-6-phosphate deficiency in African Americans (see Chapter 6, Cross-Cultural Psychopharmacology), and polymorphism of enzymes involved in psychotropic drug metabolism (Chapter 6, Cross-Cultural Psychopharmacology) are examples of important ethnic and cultural factors to be considered when assessing Axis III general medical conditions. Axis IV allows inclusion of key information from the psychosocial, environmental, and cultural domains in the assessment of stressors (see Chapter 5, Cultural Formulation). These include the following:

- Problems with the primary support group
- Problems related to the social environment
- Educational problems
- Occupational problems
- Housing problems
- Economic problems
- Problems regarding access to health care services
- Problems related to interaction with the legal system or crime
- Other psychosocial environmental problems

Different ethnic and cultural groups, including immigrants, are subjected to different stressors. Poor immigrants and migrants may be more vulnerable to certain stressors. These may be reflected in the nature of problems documented in Axis IV.

The assignment of global assessment of functioning scores involves the assessment of psychological, social, and occupational performances. These variables are likewise influenced by cultural factors and should be taken into consideration when scoring.

■ CONCLUSION

In DSM-IV there has been an attempt to include more cultural information as compared with previous editions. However, as noted in this chapter, actual information in each diagnostic category is still rather sparse, sporadic, and incomplete. More research about cultural aspects of each diagnostic category is needed.

■ REFERENCES

1. American Psychiatric Association: Diagnostic and Statistical Manual of Mental Disorders, 4th Edition, Text Revision. Washington, DC, American Psychiatric Association, 2000
2. Mezzich JE, Kleinman A, Fabrega Jr H, Parron DL (eds): Culture and Psychiatric Diagnosis. Washington, DC, American Psychiatric Press, 1996
3. Zola IK: Culture and symptoms: an analysis of patients' presenting complaints. American Sociological Review 31:615–630, 1966

■ RECOMMENDED FURTHER READING

Mezzich JE, Kleinman A, Fabrega Jr H, Parron DL (eds): Culture and Psychiatric Diagnosis. Washington, DC, American Psychiatric Press, 1996

4

CULTURE-BOUND SYNDROMES

DSM-IV-TR (1) defines culture-bound syndromes (CBSs) as "recurrent, locality-specific patterns of aberrant behavior and troubling experience . . . indigenously considered to be 'illnesses,' or at least afflictions . . . generally limited to specific societies or culture areas. . . . [They] are localized, folk, diagnostic categories that frame coherent meanings for certain repetitive, patterned, and troubling sets of experiences and observations" (1, p. 898). These include named categories in folk nosological systems, as well as "idioms of distress" or culturally salient expressions for communicating symptoms. Syndromes with names like *koro, amok, latah, pibloktoq, brain fag, falling out,* and *possession* in their local settings have been studied and reported in the psychiatric literature (2–4). These categories of illness appear to fall outside conventional Western psychiatric categories. Other categories such as obesity, anorexia nervosa, "type A behavior pattern," "petism," by virtue of their reported prevalence in Western societies, have also been suggested as Western CBSs (5).

In recent years, there has been a resurgence of interest in CBSs among clinicians, nosologists, cross-cultural psychiatrists, and anthropologists, mainly due to the increasing exposure of Western-trained clinicians to patients of diverse cultural backgrounds. This phenomenon is caused partially by increasing ease of travel and migration, changes in the way general health care and mental health care are delivered to people of various ethnic backgrounds in industrialized countries, and the need for an international classificatory system of mental illness that includes these local categories. The presentation of a CBS can be dramatic and confounding, and the clinical issues CBSs generate can be challenging, as illustrated by the following clinical vignette:

> A middle-aged Cambodian-Chinese male immigrant was admitted to a general hospital psychiatric ward in Cambridge, Massachusetts, for grossly deviant conduct in the community. He was noted to have spoken and acted bizarrely. A psychiatric consultation was requested to clarify his diagnosis and treatment. He spoke some English and the Amoy Chinese dialect. He appeared to be a soft-spoken, cooperative patient. Examination revealed that he wore a red bandanna around his head and claimed this as a way of warding off evil spirits. He mentioned that he was possessed by 13 of his relatives. He demonstrated the possession to me by crawling on the floor. The spirit possessed him at various periods of the day.

Western practitioners of mental health called to treat or consult such a case would immediately consider many clinical questions: Is the patient psychotic or schizophrenic? Is he hysterical or malingering? What are the meanings of his behavioral patterns? Why did he express his distress in such particular manners? If he feels he is "possessed," how would this diagnosis fit with existing DSM-IV or ICD-10 (6) classifications? Are his symptoms a variant of a universal psychopathological process, or are they simply a locally shaped idiom of distress? How should one treat such a patient? Is the use of psychotropic medications appropriate, and how might he respond?

These questions bring to the fore key issues in the current debate about the definition and classification of CBSs. In this chapter, I first describe the evolution of the CBS concept and provide an overview of some of the best-described syndromes. Next, I clarify the issues surrounding the current debate on the definitions and classification of CBSs. I then suggest a decision tree that would assist clinicians to differentiate CBSs from other current DSM-IV categories of mental illnesses. Finally, I propose a tentative classification of CBSs that can be integrated into the DSM-V.

■ EVOLUTION OF THE CBS CONCEPT

Early Western explorers were intrigued with manifestations of local aberrant human behavior in non-Western cultures that were considered "exotic" (7). In 1770, Captain Cook noted the condition called *amok*, a Malaysian term for a homicidal frenzy preceded by a state of brooding and ending with somnolence and amnesia. In the late nineteenth century, W. Gilmore Ellis, Superintendent of the Singapore Government Asylum, described *latah*, a condition found predominantly among Malaysians, characterized by hypersensitivity to fright marked by echopraxia, echolalia, command obedience, and dissociative or trancelike behavior. In 1895, Blonk described *koro* among Chinese living in Celebes, now Indonesia, which is characterized by the complaint of genital retraction associated with fear of resultant death. Even Emil Kraepelin in his travel in Java and India noted the diversity with which psychopathology presents itself in different cultures. He introduced the term *vergleichende psychiatrie* in 1904 to denote the study of mental illness in these different cultural groups (7).

Practitioners initially employed such terms as *ethnic neurosis* or *psychosis, exotic psychosis, psychogenic psychosis, hysterical psychosis, atypical culture-bound reactive syndrome, folk diagnostic categories,* and *culture-specific disorders.* However, the term *culture-bound syndrome,* introduced by the late Pow-Ming Yap, a Western-trained Chinese psychiatrist from Hong Kong, is best known and most widely used. DSM-IV has now officially adopted this term to describe these phenomena. Most of the current CBSs are assigned to Appendix I of DSM-IV (and its Text Revision published in 2000).

■ DESCRIPTION OF SOME OF THE BEST-KNOWN CBSs

To appreciate the issues surrounding the debate on the definition and classification of CBSs, I first describe some of the best-known CBSs (see also Appendix A, Glossary of Culture-Bound Syndromes in DSM-IV).

Koro

The term *koro* is believed to have come from a Malaysian word meaning "tortoise" (8). Terms for similar conditions include *suk-yoong, suo-yang* (China), *jinjinia bemar* (Assam), and *roo-joo* (Thailand). It is manifested by acute panic/anxiety associated with the fear of genital retraction and is accompanied by the thought that complete disappearance of the organ into the abdomen will result in death. Desperate measures are taken to prevent retraction, including applying clamps or strings and summoning friends and relatives to help. Many cases of the syndrome have been described in Southeast Asia, sometimes in epidemic proportions. There are also numerous case reports of *koro*-like states in non-Asian patients. Although the illness generally afflicts males, females describing breast and labial involution have also been reported (9). The course of the illness is usually brief, and the illness is self-limiting. *Koro* has been classified as a panic disorder, somatoform disorder, depersonalization disorder, or even psychotic disorder.

Latah

Latah is well described among the Malays and is characterized by hypersensitivity to sudden fright or startle, often with echopraxia, echolalia, command obedience, and dissociative or trancelike behavior (3). Afflicted individuals typically respond to a sudden stimulus with an exaggerated startle, sometimes dropping or throwing objects held in the hand, and often uttering obscene words. Because their behaviors are often considered funny, they may be subjected to intentional startle for the amusement of others. Other non-

Malaysian terms thought to describe similar phenomenon include *amurakh, irkunii, ikota, olan, myriachit, menkeiti, bahtschhi, imu, mali-mali, silok,* and *jumping.* Most of those with *latah* are middle-age women of low socioeconomic status. Some scholars have not considered *latah* an illness. Others, like Simons, considered *latah* reaction a culture-specific elaboration of the potential of the startle reflex (3).

Amok

Amok is a Malaysian term used to describe a syndrome characterized by homicidal frenzy preceded by brooding and followed by exhaustion and amnesia. Similar syndromes have been noted in non-Malaysian culture, for example, *cathard* in Polynesia, *pseudonite* in the Sahara, *mal de pelea* in Puerto Rico, *whitigo* among the Cree Indians, *imu* in Japan, *mirachat* in Siberia, *pibloktoq* among the polar Eskimos, *frenzied anxiety state* in Kenya, and *Whitman syndrome* in the United States (10). Afflicted individuals are usually young or middle-aged men living away from home who have recently suffered a loss or an insult, or have otherwise "lost face." Illnesses found to be associated with *amok* include epilepsy and infections such as malaria or syphilis, schizophrenia, depression, psychosis, and dissociative reactions. Most researchers emphasize the role that culture plays in the genesis of the phenomenon (11). Carr and Tan postulated that *amok* is a culturally prescribed form of violent behavior, sanctioned by Malaysian culture as a response to a highly specific set of sociocultural conditions (12). In Malaysian society, *amok* is thought to be a way of expressing aggressive impulses among people who are ordinarily conditioned to repress their anger.

In DSM-IV, *amok* is mentioned in the cultural consideration section following discussion of intermittent explosive disorder (1, p. 665). However, unlike intermittent explosive disorder, *amok* typically occurs as a single episode rather than a pattern of aggressive behavior. In many of these, dissociation is considered a dominant feature, and *amok* has been classified as a dissociative disorder.

Pibloktoq

Pibloktoq, sometimes called *arctic hysteria,* is a syndrome found among the Arctic and Subarctic Eskimos and is characterized by abrupt episodes of extreme excitement, often followed by apparent seizures and transient coma. Afflicted individuals may manifest prodromal symptoms of tiredness, depressive silences, vagueness of expression, and confusion for several days. During attacks, individuals may exhibit motor and verbal behavioral symptoms such as tearing off clothing and becoming partially or completely nude, glossolalia, fleeing, rolling in snow, jumping into water, picking up and throwing things, performing mimetic acts and engaging in choreiform movements, and coprophagia. Victims may show supernatural strength that enables them to perform the difficult and exhausting feats described above and resist restraint and capture. Following the attack, individuals may weep, manifest body tremor, feverishness, and bloodshot eyes, and have a high pulse rate. Exhausted, individuals may sleep for many hours. Afterward, rational behavior is resumed (13).

Women are more prone to *pibloktoq* than are men. Afflicted individuals are thought to be experiencing acute helplessness with panic/anxiety, and the traumatized ego is thought to react in a regressed psychological manner, albeit congruent with Eskimo ethnic culture. *Pibloktoq* was considered by earlier authors to be a hysterical phenomenon (13). In DSM-IV, *pibloktoq* is mentioned as a culturally defined "running" syndrome of dissociative fugue disorder. It should be differentiated from other syndromes that are judged to be the direct physiological consequence of a specific general medical condition, complex partial seizures, substance-induced physiological effects, mania, schizophrenia, and malingering. Hypervitaminosis A has been suggested as a possible contributing factor (14).

Brain Fag

Brain fag is a term that originated in West Africa and was originally described by Prince (4) to refer to a condition experienced by Nigerian students, primarily male, in response to the stress of their schooling. Students with this syndrome often complain that their brain is "fatigued." Now found to be widespread among South Saharan Africans, the syndrome is characterized by unpleasant head symptoms (e.g., burning, crawling sensations, vacancy feeling), visual difficulties (blurring, eye pain, excessive tearing), inability to grasp the meaning of printed symbols and sometimes of spoken words, poor retention, and fatigue and sleepiness in spite of adequate rest (4). Although *brain fag* has been compared with *neurasthenia* in Chinese, *hwa-byung* in Koreans, and *susto* in Latin Americans, many scholars considered it to be a case of anxiety/depressive or somatoform syndrome. Indeed, cases of *brain fag* have been reported to respond well to antidepressants, antianxiety medications, and relaxation therapy (4).

Shenjing Shuairuo

In Mandarin Chinese, *shenjing* means "nervous system" and *shuairuo* means "weakness." Prominent among Chinese, this condition is perceived as a weakness of the nervous system that describes a syndrome characterized by feelings of physical and mental exhaustion, difficulty concentrating, memory loss, fatigue, and dizziness. Physical complaints of difficulty sleeping, loss of appetite, sexual dysfunction, headaches, and irritability often accompany it. Known in the West as *neurasthenia, shenjing shuairuo* is officially included in the *Chinese Classification of Mental Disorders,* second edition (CCMD-2) (1, p. 902) and the *ICD-10 Classification of Mental and Behavioural Disorders.* There is an ongoing debate regarding whether *shenjing shuairuo* is actually a major depressive disorder (7).

Hwa-Byung

Hwa-byung is a Korean term that means "illness *(byung)* of fire *(hwa)*." Because "fire" corresponds to anger in Asian metaphysical thinking, *hwa byung* is an "illness of anger." The afflicted individual complains of feelings of oppression or pressure in the chest, a mass in the epigastrium or abdomen, a hot sensation pushing up in the chest, a "hot" sensation in the body, indigestion, dyspnea, fatigue, sighing, and headache. Emotional symptoms include fearfulness, panic, dysphoria, sad mood, nihilistic ideas, loss of interest, suicidal ideas, and guilt (15). The illness affects women more than men. Among Koreans, the syndrome is thought to be related to suppression of chronic anger and indignation.

Hwa-byung has been compared to DSM-III categories of major depression, somatization disorder, generalized anxiety disorder, and obsessive-compulsive disorder (15).

Ataque de Nervios

Ataque de nervios, or "attack of nerves," is a popular illness among Puerto Ricans and other Latinos. It refers to a culturally sanctioned response to acute stressful experiences, particularly relating to grief during funerals, to threat, at the scene of an accident, and during a family conflict (16). It is characterized by uncontrollable shouting, trembling, heart palpitations, a sense of heat in the chest rising to the head, fainting, and seizurelike activities. Consciousness is regained quickly, with amnesia of the episode. Afflicted individuals are likely to be female, over age 45 with less than a high school education, and socially disadvantaged. *Ataque de nervios* has been found to likely meet Western criteria for depression, dysthymia, generalized anxiety disorder, panic disorder, and posttraumatic stress disorder (16).

Taijin Kyofusho

Taijin kyofusho, found among the Japanese, is also referred to as "anthropophobia" (7). The term *taijin* refers to "interpersonal," and *kyofusho* means "phobia" or "fear." Afflicted individuals report that their bodies, body parts, or body functions may offend, embarrass, or displease others. Symptoms include fear of embarrassing others by blushing; of causing discomfort by one's gaze, facial expression, or body odor; or of offending others by speaking one's thoughts aloud (7). The disorder primarily affects young people. Symptoms are most prominent in interpersonal situations. Indeed, in DSM-IV *taijin kyofusho* is considered to be a social phobia. The higher prevalence among Japanese may be related to cultural values that emphasizes the importance of proper behavior in all social situations.

Possession Disorder

Capranzano defined possession as "any altered state of consciousness indigenously interpreted in terms of the influence of an alien spirit" (17). The phenomenon of possession has been reported worldwide. Possession states are often accepted as normal when they occur in the context of a broadly accepted collective cultural or religious practice. Alternatively, these experiences can be regarded as abnormal, particularly when possessed individuals become so distressed and dysfunctional that they seek assistance from healers and physicians. Possession states in different cultures have included *amok* and *bebainan* (Indonesia), *latah* (Malaysia), *pibloktoq* (Arctic), *ataque de nervios* (Latin America), and *zar* (North Africa and Middle East). Possessed individuals often report the experience of "being possessed" by another entity, such as a person, god, demon, animal, or inanimate object. Usual complaints involve single or episodic disturbances of consciousness, identity, or memory. Symptoms of loss of control over one's action, loss of awareness of one's surrounding, or loss of one's identity; change in tone of voice; and loss of perceived sensitivity to pain often are associated with the complaint of possession. Possession affects women more than men. Affected individuals are often from lower socioeconomic levels and educational backgrounds (17).

In DSM-IV-TR, pathological possession is placed in the category of dissociative trance disorder under dissociative disorder not otherwise specified (1, p. 784). Possession should be differentiated from other dissociative disorders, acute distress disorder, posttraumatic stress disorder, somatization disorder, complex partial seizures, psychotic disorders, and disorders associated with a general medical condition.

■ CLARIFYING THE DEFINITION OF A CULTURE-BOUND SYNDROME

Ever since the introduction of the term *culture-bound syndrome,* scholars have debated the precise definition and utility of the term. As originally conceptualized by Yap (2), a CBS connotes the following concepts:

1. It is primarily a *psychological* process whereby "mental experience brings about an abnormal reaction in a predisposed subject. The predisposition may be conceived in wholly or partly somatic terms" (2, p. 34).

2. It is *reactive* in that "an abnormal reaction has been produced by an external traumatic shock of great severity in a mechanical manner or has been brought into open expression in a predisposed subject by an external, experiential stress" (2, p. 34).

3. It is *severe,* almost reaching a "psychotic" degree of disturbance of psychic functioning. Disturbance may involve "loss of insight, loss of contact with reality, significant impairment of the ability to understand and use language, loss of control over instinctual life, and dramatic change in the whole personality and impairment of adaptive powers" (2, pp. 34–35).

Yap's original classification emphasized diagnosis based on the syndrome. Yap defined CBSs as "forms of psychopathology produced by [a] certain system of implicit values, social structure and obviously shared beliefs indigenous to certain areas" (2, p. 38). He considered CBSs to be atypical variants of generally distributed Western psychogenic disorders. Yap considered them "culture-bound" because "their *symptom patterns* are unusual and are determined by cultural factors in both *form* and *frequency.*" Even though diverse links are traceable between the illness and its sociocultural background for all CBSs, Yap cautioned against overgeneralization about the relationship between culture and mental illness from the material available. He argued that CBSs are neither rare nor "exotic" and suggested that the atypical presentation of some CBSs merely reflects variation in specific cultural forms and social structure (2).

Based on key syndromal features, Yap suggested two ways of understanding the CBS: 1) as a variant or "atypical" form of existing prototype of mental illness, and 2) as an "atypical" pattern of paranoia or emotional or disordered consciousness.

In the first category, CBSs (denoted below by quotation marks) were viewed as atypical forms of typical prototypes of affective and dissociative disorders:

1. Primary fear reaction

   - Acute anxiety and panic: "malignant anxiety"
   - States of hypersuggestibility: "*latah* reaction"
   - Traumatic anxiety/depressive states: "*susto*"
   - Severe psychophysiological reaction to terror: "psychogenic death"

2. Hypereridic (undifferentiated morbid hostile) rage reaction

   - Acute psychopathic reaction: "*amok*"

3. Specific, culturally imposed nosophobia

   - Depersonalization states with severe anxiety: "*koro*"

4. Trance dissociation

   - "*Windigo*" and "*hsieh-ping*" (2, p. 41)

In the second category, CBSs are tentatively classified as follows:

1. Paranoid syndrome
2. Emotional syndrome

   - Depersonalization state: "*koro*"
   - Fear-induced depressive state: "*susto*"

3. Syndrome of disordered consciousness

   - Impaired consciousness: "*latah* reaction"
   - Turbid states: malignant anxiety, "*amok*," "*negi-negi*"

- Dissociated consciousness: certain types of possession syndrome, *"hsieh-ping," "windigo"* psychosis (2, p. 42)

Whereas many CBSs arguably cannot be considered "psychotic," most cross-cultural psychiatrists would generally agree on classification of CBSs based on a syndrome that is akin to classification of diseases of general medical conditions based on symptoms and signs. However, across disciplines and among researchers, there remains no clear consensus on the definition of CBSs. Considerable confusion currently exists in the usage of this term.

Current debate about the definition of CBSs generally falls within two camps:

1. The syndromal approach: CBSs are variants of a universal disease process with emphasis on diagnosis based on syndromal patterns (2–4).
2. The meaning-centered approach: CBSs are uniquely locally shaped cultural expression of "illness" that defy inclusion in current Western categories of mental illness (18).

Syndromal Approach

The syndromal approach conforms closely to the current DSM-IV classificatory scheme and is favored by many cross-cultural psychiatrists. Proponents of this viewpoint emphasize a more traditional biomedical approach that searches for a physiological substrate in the pathogenesis of CBSs. CBSs are defined by syndrome, an aggregate of signs and symptoms associated with any morbid process that together constitute the picture of the disease (not including notions of cause) and is restricted to a limited number of cultures by reason of certain of their psychosocial features (4). This view assumes that CBSs are manifestations of a set of universal categories of psychopathology uniquely shaped by specific cultural forms and social structures. These categories should be subsumed under present Western psychiatric nosology (2). Proponents of the syndromal approach generally agree with Yap, who cautioned against the proliferation of diagnostic categories that eventually may be found to have common physiological substrates. Although not ignoring the shaping influence of sociocultural factors in disease etiology, a syndromal approach gives preeminence to presumed physiological factors.

An example of the syndromal approach is Simons and Hughes's proposal of sorting of CBSs into different *taxa*, a term borrowed from biology to denote a tentative grouping of behavioral characteristics based on similarity without specifying the level of abstraction (3). Depending on the key defining behavioral patterns and the strength of their scientific evidences, they sorted CBSs into the following taxa:

1. Those with some evidence to support the hypothesis of a neurophysiological shaping factor

   - The startle matching taxon: *latah*
   - The sleep paralysis taxon: *uquamairineq*, "old hag" phenomenon

2. Those with a suspected neurophysiological shaping factor

   - The genital retraction taxon: *koro*
   - The sudden mass assault taxon: *amok*
   - The running taxon: *pibloktoq* among the polar Eskimos, *grisi siknis* in Miskito culture

3. Those that should probably no longer be considered because of insufficient verifiable clinical evidence or presumed attributed etiological significance

   - The fright illness taxon: *susto* among Hispanics; *saladera,* a misfortune syndrome among the Peruvian Amazon culture; *lanti* among Visayan Filipinos; and *mogo laya,* a New Guinea fright illness
   - The cannibal compulsion taxon: *windigo* psychosis among the Northern Algonkian people (3)

Meaning-Centered Approach

Ritenbaugh and Cassidy have proposed broadening the definition of CBSs to be applicable in all cultures to varying degrees rather than in the narrow sense that has been used historically. They include notions of etiology and treatment and define a CBS as a constellation of symptoms that together have been categorized as a dysfunction or disease (18). Their definition of a CBS includes the following characteristics:

- It cannot be understood apart from its specific cultural or subcultural context
- The etiology summarizes and symbolizes core meanings and behavioral norms of that culture
- Diagnosis relies on culture-specific technology as well as ideology
- Successful treatment is accomplished only by participants in that culture (18)

According to Ritenbaugh and Cassidy, symptoms of CBSs may be recognized and similarly organized elsewhere but are not categorized as the same dysfunction or "disease." Treatment judged as successful in one cultural context may not be understood as successful from another perspective.

Proponents of a meaning-centered approach, generally favored by some anthropologists, criticize biomedicine for its failure to recognize culture and its exclusion of culture in its basic explanatory model, which has been developed within Western cultures and within the biomedical system. They are concerned that a redefinition of syndromes from other cultures into current Western biomedical terms may leave out potentially important cultural patterns relevant to diagnosis or treatment. By subsuming all diseases in all cultures under a broader definition of CBSs, a clarifying focus may hopefully be provided that will also subject biomedicine to critical analysis (18).

Although intended to be more inclusive of cultural variables in the examination and understanding of illness categories, a meaning-centered diagnostic scheme unfortunately led to a proliferation of conditions, which generated more confusion for clinicians. Categories such as mild to moderate obesity (18), protein-energy malnutrition *(kwashiorkor)* (19), the type A behavior of coronary-prone individuals (20), premenstrual syndrome (21), and adolescence in American society (22) have been proposed under this broadened definition of CBSs, which rendered the usage of the term *CBS* meaningless. Nonetheless, aberrant patterns of behavior outside the Western classification of psychiatric disorders do exist throughout the world. The concern of including a cultural variable in clinical care and research endeavor is a point well taken. Four epidemics of *koro* disorder have been reported in the past decade (11). Yet, for most Western clinicians, conditions such as *koro* still defy classification in the current Western nosological system. As a result, research on and treatment of such conditions remains unclear, unfocused, and understudied.

Further confusing the diagnostic issue is that the current definition of the term *CBS* also includes categories of "illness of attribution" (i.e., illness defined not by specific signs and symptoms but by real or presumed causes such as the emotion of fear or anger, an outside supernatural force such as witchcraft or possession, or an organic disturbance such as "bad blood" or semen loss) (7). An example is *susto,* a folk diagnosis used in Latin American countries to describe a variety of ailments attributed to an antecedent fright or startle.

Although many have suggested that illnesses of attribution be excluded from categories of CBSs because they are not true syndromes, it is important for Western mental health practitioners to be aware of and understand these non-Western notions of etiology. In the cultures in which they are found, they are highly prevalent. They constitute an integral part of the folk experience of illness and healing. With the current interest in alternative medicine and care, it behooves Western clinicians to understand such notions of illness and to consider how to integrate these insights into Western approaches of delivering care so that mental health services may be perceived as more culturally congruent.

One further confounding factor in the understanding of CBSs is that the criteria of "culture specificity" have not been clearly defined. Although Levine and I have proposed criteria of culture specificity (11), such criteria have not been generally accepted. The criteria of the concept of culture specificity is elaborated on later in this chapter.

■ CLASSIFICATIONS OF CBSs IN DSM AND ICD

Given the current status of CBSs, how could they be eventually incorporated into future volumes of DSM and ICD? I suggest the following process:

1. *Mapping out the essential features of CBSs.* A scientific study of CBSs should begin with a careful description and analysis of the signs and symptoms of each CBS, such as in the study by Simons on the syndromal patterns of *latah* (23). Without clear delineation of signs and symptoms, clinicians would be at a loss to recognize patterns of aberrant behavior that signal the presence of a CBS. Differentiation of CBSs from other behavioral disorders would be difficult. Potential biological factors that may underlie CBSs would be missed.
2. *Translations of local names to English.* To avoid the confusion of the multiplicity of names that have been used to describe various CBSs, the use of local names should be avoided as much as possible. Hughes's (3) organization of each CBS under the following four headings is a good start for comparative study:

   - Alternative spellings of syndrome names
   - Label according to source group's geographic locale or the cultural context of the term if geographic localization would not be sufficiently specific (e.g., "Hispanic cultures")
   - Symptoms commonly reported and/or discussions of the syndrome
   - Important literature references

As a sample entry, Hughes (5) cited *amok* as follows:

A. *ahade idizi be* (Newman 1964); *cafard* (Yap 1951, p. 319); *cathard* (Kiev 1972, p. 86); *soudonite* (Kiev 1972, p. 86; Yap 1951, p. 319); *mal de pelea* (Rothenberg 1964; Yap 1974, p. 98); *colera* (Yap 1974, p. 98); *ngamok* (Schmidt 1964, p. 148); *gila besi* (Schmidt 1964, p. 149)
B. Malaysia, Indonesia
C. Dissociative episode(s); outburst(s) of violence and aggressive or homicidal behavior directed at people and objects; persecutory ideas; automatism; amnesia; exhaustion and return to consciousness following the episode (for *amok* runners who are not killed during the episode)
D. Kiev (1972); Murphy (1973); Teoh (1972); van Loon (1926/1927); van Wulfften Palthe (1936, pp. 529–531); Yap (1974); and chapters by Arboleda-Florez, Burton-Bradley, Carr, and Westermeyer in Simons and Hughes (1985, p. 77)

3. *Classify CBSs using current DSM categories and with descriptive criteria.* There are enough entries in the current DSM-IV diagnostic system to allow CBSs to be classified. In considering the various ways in which CBSs can be designated within DSM-IV, it is important to attend to the criteria set for each DSM-IV diagnostic category. Categories subsumed under "illness of attribution" and "idiom of distress" should be excluded (7). Because the criteria set for most of the current CBSs do not as yet reach the threshold of the current standards for inclusion into the main text of DSM-IV, coding of most CBSs could be classified according to one of the following suggested DSM-IV schemes (1, p. 5):

- V codes (for other conditions that may be a focus of clinical attention)
- Diagnosis or condition deferred
- Unspecified mental disorder (nonpsychotic)

- Disorders not otherwise specified (NOS)

For most CBSs, the disorders NOS category should apply. DSM-IV allows for inclusion of the NOS category in the following four situations (1, p. 4):

- The presentation conforms to the general guidelines for a mental disorder in the diagnostic class, but the symptomatic picture does not meet criteria for any of the specific disorders.
- The presentation conforms to a symptom pattern that has not been included in the DSM-IV Classification but that causes clinically significant distress or impairment. Research criteria for some of these symptom patterns have been included in Appendix B of the DSM-IV.
- There is uncertainty about etiology (i.e., whether the disorder is due to a general medical condition, is substance-induced, or is primary).
- There is insufficient opportunity for complete data collection (e.g., in an emergency situation) or inconsistent or contradictory information, but there is enough information to place it within a particular diagnostic class (e.g., the clinician determines that the individual has psychotic symptoms but does not have enough information to diagnose a specific psychotic disorder).

When aggregate data on CBSs reach the scientific threshold as verified by field testing and experts' consensus opinion, then CBSs should be included in the main body of each of the current DSM-IV nosological categories.

Eventually, many current categories of CBSs can be classified in DSM-IV under the following disorder NOS headings:

- Brief reactive psychosis (298.80)
- Atypical psychosis (298.80)
- Social phobia (300.23)
- Atypical anxiety disorder (300.00)
- Atypical somatoform disorder (300.71)
- Depersonalization disorder (300.60)

- Factitious disorder with psychological symptoms (300.16)
- Intermittent [isolated] explosive disorder (312.35) (3, p. 15)

4. *Define the context of the CBSs experience.* Sociocultural variables and the context of the occurrence of CBSs should be captured and explicated. Some CBSs have occurred as isolated cases (orphaned cases), some have occurred in epidemic proportion. Without spelling out the context of its occurrence, important sociocultural variables would be missed in the understanding of the pathogenesis of the CBSs. Decontexualized CBSs become clinically sterile. Much would be lost if psychiatric entities were not enriched by findings from anthropological researches. Systematic entry of the context of the illness experience could be included in the description of psychosocial variables in the current DSM-IV Axis IV.

5. *Agreement on culture-specific criteria.* Consideration should be given to what constitutes "culture-specific criteria." Bernstein (11) and I suggest the following:

   - The disorder must be a discrete, well-defined syndrome.
   - It must be recognized as a specific illness in the culture with which it is primarily associated.
   - The disorder must be expected, recognized, and to some degree sanctioned as a response to certain precipitants in the particular culture.
   - A higher incidence or prevalence of the disorder must exist in societies in which the disorder is culturally recognized, compared with other societies.

   Adherence to these criteria would encourage and allow integration of anthropological and epidemiological data into CBS categories and aid in differential diagnosis.

6. *Adherence to a decision tree for the diagnosis of CBSs.* Figure 4–1 is a decision tree for CBSs proposed by Levine and myself (11) that we feel would be useful for clinicians in consideration of differential diagnosis of CBSs with current DSM-IV categories. CBSs should be reserved only for those syndromes that meet culture-specific criteria.

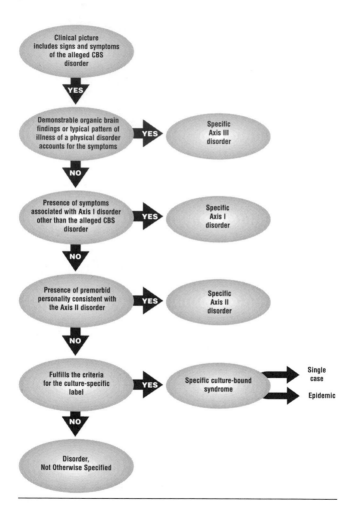

FIGURE 4–1. **Proposed decision tree for culture-bound syndromes (CBSs) in DSM-IV.**

■ PROPOSAL FOR A CLASSIFICATION OF CBSs IN DSM-IV

To be consistent with DSM-IV's emphasis on classification of each syndrome based on a criteria set, several of the better-known and better-studied CBSs could be classified in the DSM-IV under the NOS category with qualifying features:

Dissociative Disorder NOS

Dissociation is a disruption in the usually integrated functions of consciousness, memory, identity, or perception of the environment. The disturbance may be sudden or gradual, transient or chronic. In several of the CBSs, dissociation is a prominent feature. As noted by Spiegel and Cardena, "nowhere should cultural influences on symptomatology be more noticeable than among the dissociative disorders that can be understood as extreme and dramatic responses to behavior or socially induced trauma. Thus the content of dissociative symptoms and to some extent the process of dissociative disorders reflect the diversity of cultures, although the mental mechanisms underlying these symptoms may be presumed to be universal" (24).

- Dissociative disorder NOS with features of startle matching: *latah*
- Dissociative disorder NOS with features of fugue reaction: *pibloktoq* (Arctic Eskimo), *grisi siknis* (Miskito Indian)
- Dissociative disorder NOS with features of identity disorder: *possession* disorder, *shin-byung* (Korean)

If the development of characteristic anxiety, dissociative, and other symptoms occurred within 1 month after the exposure to an extreme traumatic stressor and lasted from 2 days to 4 weeks, the above examples could also be classified as acute stress disorder NOS.

Acute Stress Disorder NOS

- Acute Stress Disorder NOS with features of conversion reaction: *falling out* (African American, Caribbean)
- Anxiety disorder NOS: *ataque de nervios* (Latinos)
- Social phobia NOS: *taijin kyofusho* (Japan)
- Panic disorder NOS with fear of capsizing or drowning: *kayak angst* (Inuit Eskimo)

Somatoform Disorder NOS

- Somatoform disorder NOS with features of fatigue: *brain fag* (West Africa), neurasthenia (Western countries), *shenjing shuairuo* (Chinese), chronic fatigue syndrome (Western countries)
- Atypical somatoform disorder NOS with features of genital retraction and panic reaction: *koro* (China, Thailand, Singapore, India, Indonesia, Malaysia) (An alternative to this classification would be panic/anxiety disorder NOS with features of genital retraction.)

Intermittent Explosive Disorder NOS

- Intermittent explosive disorder NOS with features of mass assault: *amok*

As an example, the case vignette mentioned earlier in the chapter (assuming the case turned out to be a case of possession syndrome) can be classified as follows:

Axis I: 300.15 dissociative disorder NOS with possession features
Axis II: Deferred
Axis III: Deferred
Axis IV: Degree of stress: moderate; psychosocial stressors: unclear at present
Axis V: GAF: on admission = 30; current = 45

■ CONCLUSION

Since its inception, scholars have struggled with the concept of CBSs. The struggle is reflected in the current application of the term to describe a variety of illnesses that are presumed to be shaped by local culture. Most authors would agree that the term *culture-bound syndrome* was intended to describe forms of otherwise common mental illness that are rendered unusual because of the shaping influence of culture on behavior. The dialectical debate of the conceptualization of CBSs emphasizing either biological or sociocultural influence should be avoided. I believe that an integrated biopsychosocial approach that includes important sociocultural variables offers the best paradigm in understanding CBSs. CBSs offer an opportunity to study mental illnesses in their natural settings. Because they are eloquent examples of the influence of culture on psychopathology, they are superb models for examining the interplay between psychological, social, cultural, and biological contributions to mental illness. By elucidating the "bio-psycho-social-cultural" mechanisms of those afflicted with these syndromes, we may better recognize the interplay of these mechanisms within all kinds of psychopathology.

■ REFERENCES

1. American Psychiatric Association: Diagnostic and Statistical Manual of Mental Disorders, 4th Edition, Text Revision. Washington, DC, American Psychiatric Association, 2000
2. Yap PM: The culture-bound reactive syndromes, in Mental Health Research in Asia and the Pacific. Edited by Caudill W, Lin TY. Honolulu, HI, East-West Center Press, 1969, pp 33–53
3. Simons RC, Hughes CC (eds): The Culture-Bound Syndromes. Dordrecht, Netherlands, Reidel, 1985
4. Prince R: The concept of culture-bound syndromes: anorexia nervosa and brain-fag. Soc Sci Med 21:197–203, 1985

5. Simons RC, Hughes CC (eds): Culture-bound syndromes, in Culture, Ethnicity, and Mental Illness. Edited by Gaw AC. Washington, DC, American Psychiatric Press, 1993, pp 75–99

6. World Health Organization: International Statistical Classification of Diseases and Related Health Problems, 10th Revision. Geneva, World Health Organization, 1992

7. Levine RE, Gaw AC: Culture-bound syndromes. Psychiatr ClinNorth Am 18:523–536, 1995

8. Yap PM: Koro: a culture-bound depersonalization syndrome. Br J Psychiatry 111:43–50, 1965

9. Bernstein RL, Gaw AC: Koro: proposed classification for DSM-IV. Am J Psychiatry 147:1670–1674, 1990

10. Carr JE: Ethnobehaviorism and the culture-bound syndromes: the case of amok, in The Culture-Bound Syndromes. Edited by Simons RC, Hughes CC. Dordrecht, Netherlands, Reidel, 1985, pp 199–223

11. Gaw AC, Bernstein RL: Classification of amok in the DSM-IV. Hospital and Community Psychiatry 43:789–793, 1992

12. Carr JE, Tan EK: In search of the true amok: amok as viewed within the Malay culture. Am J Psychiatry 133:1295–1299, 1976

13. Gussow Z: Pibloktoq (hysteria) among the polar Eskimo, in The Culture-Bound Syndromes. Edited by Simons RC, Hughes CC. Dordrecht, Netherlands, Reidel, 1985, pp 271–287

14. Landy D: Pibloktoq (hysteria) and Inuit nutrition: possible implication of hypervitaminosis A. Soc Sci Med 21:173–185, 1985

15. Kim LIC: Psychiatric care of Korean Americans, in Culture, Ethnicity and Mental Illness. Edited by Gaw AC. Washington, DC, American Psychiatric Press, 1993, pp 347–375

16. Guarnaccia PJ: Ataque de nervios in Puerto Rico: culture-bound syndrome or popular illness? Med Anthropol 15:157–170, 1993

17. Gaw AC, Ding Q, Levine RE, et al: The clinical characteristics of possession disorder among 20 Chinese patients in the Hebei Province of China. Psychiatr Serv 49:360–365, 1998

18. Ritenbaugh C: Obesity as a culture-bound syndrome. Cult Med Psychiatry 6:347–361, 1982
19. Cassidy CM: Protein-energy malnutrition as a culture-bound syndrome. Cult Med Psychiatry 6:325–345, 1982
20. Helman CG: Heart disease and the cultural construction of time: the type A behavior pattern as a Western culture-bound syndrome. Soc Sci Med 25:969–979, 1987
21. Johnson TM: Premenstrual syndrome as a Western culture-specific disorder. Cult Med Psychiatry 11:337–356, 1987
22. Hill RF, Fortenberry DJ: Adolescence as a culture-bound syndrome. Soc Sci Med 35:73–80, 1992
23. Spiegel D, Cardena E: Cultural diversity of dissociative and somatoform disorders. Paper presented at the NIMH Conference on Culture and Diagnosis, Pittsburgh, PA, April 1991
24. Simons RC: The resolution of the Latah paradox. Journal of Nervous and Mental Illness 168:195–206, 1980

■ RECOMMENDED FURTHER READING

American Psychiatric Association: Appendix I: outline for cultural formulation and glossary of culture-bound syndromes, in Diagnostic and Statistical Manual of Mental Disorders, 4th Edition, Text Revision. Washington, DC, American Psychiatric Association, 2000, pp 897–903 (see also Appendix A, Glossary of Culture-Bound Syndromes in DSM-IV, and Table 5–1 in this volume)

Simons RC, Hughes CC (eds): Culture-bound syndromes, in Culture, Ethnicity, and Mental Illness. Edited by Gaw AC. Washington, DC, American Psychiatric Press, 1993, pp 75–99

5

CULTURAL FORMULATION

Cultural formulation (CF) is a set of guidelines that clinicians use as a cultural analysis process that relates to every clinical encounter (1). Its purpose is to assist the clinician in systematically evaluating and reporting the impact of the individual's cultural context in the illness experience. By applying a cultural perspective to the clinical interview process, clinicians can elucidate an objective picture of the context of the experience of the patient's particular episode of illness that one hopes will lend greater clarity and coherence to the formulation of a psychiatric diagnosis and treatment plan. Judgment on "normality or abnormality" of an individual's behavior can be inferred by the degree of deviation of that particular behavior from the individual's own larger sociocultural milieu. Finally, by focusing on elucidation of data strictly from the patient's point of view, CF guidelines can help to prevent clinicians from injecting their personal biases into the interview.

In this chapter, I discuss the application of CF as proposed by the Cultural Task Groups of DSM-IV (2). This discussion takes the application of DSM-IV's CF one step further by explicating the technique of elucidating cultural information during a routine psychiatric interview. A clinical case is provided at the end of this chapter to illustrate the application of CF in psychiatric diagnosis and treatment.

To effectively use CF in the interview process, the interviewer should first be familiar with the following information:

1. DSM-IV multiaxial assessment
2. DSM-IV outline of CF
3. Biopsychosocial approach in patient care
4. Associative technique of interviewing

■ CF AND DSM-IV MULTIAXIAL ASSESSMENTS

In DSM-IV, CF is constructed to obtain pertinent personal and narrative cultural data that complements the manual's current five multiaxial assessments (1). Rather than having a separate "cultural axis," the interviewer is encouraged to use a *narrative description* to systematically capture relevant cultural data in each of the following DSM-IV's four axes (Axis V is for the Global Assessment of Functioning):

Axis I	Clinical disorders
	Other conditions that may be a focus of clinical attention
Axis II	Personality disorders
	Mental retardation
Axis III	General medical conditions
Axis IV	Psychosocial and environmental problems

Guidelines for CF have been provided in Appendix I of DSM-IV (see Table 5–1). The outline is designed to provide a systematic review of a patient life's experience in the following areas:

1. The individual's cultural background
2. The role of the cultural context in the expression and evaluation of symptoms and dysfunction
3. The effect those cultural differences may have on the relationship between the individual and the clinician

Given the myriad information that may constitute the individual's context of experience, how does one determine which cultural information is pertinent to pursue in the interview? For this matter, the reader is referred to articles by Lu and colleagues (3), Gaw (4),

---

TABLE 5–1. **Outline for cultural formulation in DSM-IV**

Cultural identity of the individual. Note the individual's ethnic or cultural reference groups. For immigrant and ethnic minorities, note separately the degree of involvement with both the culture of origin and the host culture (where applicable). Also note language abilities, use, and preferences (multilingualism).

Cultural explanations of the individual's illness. The following may be identified: the predominant idioms of distress through which symptoms or the need for social support are communicated (e.g., "nerves," possessing spirits, somatic complaints, inexplicable misfortune), the meaning and perceived severity of the individual's symptoms in relation to norms of the cultural reference group, any local illness category used by the individual's family and community to identify the condition, the perceived causes or explanatory models that the individual and the reference group use to explain the illness, or current preferences for and past experiences with professional and popular sources of care.

Cultural factors related to psychosocial environment and levels of functioning. Note culturally relevant interpretations of social stressors, available social supports, and levels of functioning and disability. This would include stresses in the local social environment and the role of religion and kin networks in providing emotional, instrumental, and informational support.

Cultural elements of the relationship between the individual and the clinician. Indicate differences in culture and social status between the individual and the clinician and problems that these differences may cause in diagnosis and treatment (e.g., difficulty in communicating in the individual's first language, in eliciting symptoms or understanding their cultural significance, in negotiating an appropriate relationship or level of intimacy, in determining whether a behavior is normative or pathological).

Overall cultural assessment for diagnosis and care. The formulation concludes with a discussion of how cultural considerations specifically influence comprehensive diagnosis and care.

Source. Reprinted with permission from American Psychiatric Association: *Diagnostic and Statistical Manual of Mental Illness,* 4th Edition, Text Revision. Washington, DC, American Psychiatric Association, 2000, pp. 897–898.

Mezzich and colleagues (5), and Tseng and Streltzer (6) that document and clarify how cultural factors influence the emergence, expression, and course of mental disorders and their treatment. Additionally, Lu and colleagues (3) have also provided an excellent elaboration of the content of the CF to guide clinicians in its usage. Many case examples on the application of CF have accumulated in the literature (1). Most important, keeping in mind the following DSM-IV definition of mental disorder can help the interviewer to stay focused on aspects of the history-taking in which cultural data may be explored:

> In DSM-IV, each of the mental disorders is conceptualized as a clinically significant behavioral or psychological syndrome or pattern that occurs in an individual and that is associated with present distress (e.g., a painful symptom) or disability (i.e., impairment in one or more important areas of functioning) or with a significantly increased risk of suffering death, pain, disability, or an important loss of freedom. (2, p. xxxi)

Thus, *all cultural factors that may lead to distress, disability, dysfunction, pain, suffering, loss of freedom, or death* are pertinent areas for a psychiatric inquiry. As Engel has pointed out, symptoms may emerge from disruption of the homeostasis of an individual's biological, psychological, social, or cultural level of integration (7). Disruption of the sociocultural system of integration may lead to conflicts and stresses that result in symptoms and are pertinent areas of inquiry. Scientific inquiry into cultural history requires a rigorous clinical application of the biopsychosocial approach to health and disease. Thus, rather than simply adopting a pure biomedical model, it is essential that the clinician has a good grasp of the biopsychosocial model of health and disease.

■ THE BIOPSYCHOSOCIAL APPROACH IN THE CLINICAL INTERVIEW

A biopsychosocial approach offers a comprehensive and integrated framework for health and disease (7, 8). In this approach, the clinician's attention is directed to both the biological aberration that is the characterization of the nature of the pathological processes (disease) and the symbolic element of the pathological processes, commonly referred to as *illness experience* (9). Because the illness experience is molded and influenced by the unique sociocultural experience of the individual (9, 10), its exploration provides useful cultural data.

Let us consider two clinical vignettes. The first pertains to the experience of a Caucasian patient who was raised in the United States:

A middle-aged male Caucasian presents with an Axis I diagnosis of major depression associated with chronic alcoholism and with concomitant Axis III findings of early liver cirrhosis. The interview revealed that the depression began after the recent death of his father. The father had high expectations for his son to be able to "hold a job, have a family, and lead a productive life as a member of U.S. society." The patient felt he had failed his father miserably because alcoholism (disease) had prevented him from living up to his father's expectations. He blames himself and has developed a suicidal depression.

This history contains several leads to potential cultural data that could shed light on the pathogenesis of a suicidal depression. One area that needs clarification is the relationship between father and son and how their unique cultural background may have molded this relationship. Another area is their mutual expectation and their own concept of what constitutes a "successful" life. And finally, it is important to find out how the son's alcoholism may have thwarted the fulfillment of their mutual expectation. Inquiry into this whole area of the patient's experience of illness, apart from the liver damage that may be caused by alcohol (the disease), may shed light not only on the conflict and stresses that brought on his depression, but also may provide an important linkage to the cultural matrix that gives meaning to his experience.

The second vignette pertains to the illness experience of a Chinese-speaking U.S. immigrant in Boston. This case, in contrast to the first vignette, offers a sharper presentation of cultural conflict, stresses, and symptoms:

> A Chinese-speaking U.S. immigrant, who had immigrated to Boston and worked in a Chinese restaurant, presented with a chief complaint of genital retraction and eventual fear of death, which are classic symptoms of the culture-bound syndrome *koro* (11). Although no actual death from *koro* has ever been reported, those who believe in this folk illness consider it to be fatal (11).
>
> The patient has had a long history of masturbation since his teenage years in China. He had been warned not to masturbate excessively to avoid development of *koro*. The patient reported that as long as his masturbatory activity stays within the perceived boundary of cultural tolerance he remains symptom free.
>
> On the way home one wintry day following a visit to a prostitute, the patient thought he had caught "cold." Over the course of the next few days he developed pain in his penis, which began to alarm him. To reassure himself that he had not contracted *koro,* he continued to masturbate. When on one occasion he could not obtain an erection, he panicked, thinking he might have developed the syndrome. His suspicion was reinforced when he consulted elders in Boston's Chinatown and was told he was one in 10,000 individuals who had developed *koro* and that he would die. This information plunged him into a severe depression. He could not sleep or work and had to consult many physicians. The patient twice sought emergency care and was found to have no physical or laboratory findings to corroborate a physical cause for his penile pain. Despite absence of physical findings, he was given analgesics, tranquilizers, and eventually an antibiotic, all of which were unable to relieve his pain. Because of the progression of his illness and the development of suicidal ideation, he was eventually referred for a psychiatric evaluation.

This clinical vignette offers a view of the rich interplay between sociocultural, psychological, and biological factors in the genesis of the patient's symptoms. In interviewing such a patient, it is essential to assess all clinical aspects of depression including suicidal risk and the social antecedents of the illness. Moreover, alerted to the existence of a clinical entity called *koro,* the clinician will not readily dismiss the complaints as mere symptoms of a major depressive disorder, a psychotic disorder, or even a panic/anxiety disorder (indeed, the proper classification of culture-bound syndromes such as *koro* in DSM-IV remains unresolved [11]). Furthermore, to obtain a clearer understanding of the influence of cultural background in the pathogenesis of this culture-bound syndrome, it is crucial to carefully inquire as to the sequence of the genesis of the patient's symptoms, his own belief concerning what is afflicting him, the sociocultural environment in which he grew up, and the social interaction that reinforced his fear of *koro.*

These two cases illustrate the areas of cultural inquiry to pursue in a clinical interview. The question is how to systematically elicit cultural data during the process of obtaining a clinical history.

In the course of a psychiatric interview, pertinent cultural data may be related to each of the following areas of a person's clinical history:

1. *Present illness.* All recent changes in health that led to seeking psychiatric attention
2. *Past health.* All changes in general health prior to the present illness
3. *Family health.* Health status of the entire family
4. *Personal and social history.* Information on the development, life experiences, and personal relationships of the individual that may be related to the current complaints (12)

Morgan and Engel (12) have recommended that any symptom should be fully explored in the following seven dimensions:

1. *Body location.* Where is the symptom located?
2. *Quality.* What is the symptom like?
3. *Quantity.* How intense is the symptom?
4. *Chronology.* When did the symptom begin and what course has it followed?

5. *Setting.* Under what circumstances does the symptom take place?
6. *Aggravating and alleviating factors.* What makes the symptom worse or better?
7. *Associated manifestations.* What other symptoms or phenomena are associated with it?

Such questions should be pursued for both somatic and psychological complaints. As details of symptoms are explored in depth, one is constantly alerted to possible sources of the patient's own ideas, beliefs, values, rituals, and operating procedures that may contribute to such complaints. An objective exploration of all cultural antecedents leading to the symptoms and events can be obtained through mastery of the technique of an *associative interview.*

■ ASSOCIATIVE INTERVIEW

In an *associative interview,* the patient is encouraged to continuously speak freely while the interviewer subtly provides direction during the course of interview (10). The interviewer always initiates the inquiry into each new area of the patient's history with open-ended (nondirective) questions and by following with progressively more specific (directive) questions until the subject is fully clarified. Open-ended questions such as "Tell me more about your sadness," and "What was it like to feel abandoned?" prompt the patient to elaborate. Closed-ended questioning such as "Did you feel sad?" "Were you angry when you feel abandoned?" usually elicit a "Yes" or "No" response. By starting with open-ended questioning, one avoids premature closure of the interview and limiting of important information.

The use of an associative technique is important for two reasons: 1) it allows information to flow naturally from the patient, thereby avoiding the injection of the interviewer's biases, and 2) it conveys to the patient that all information is relevant to his or her illness.

At the beginning of the interview, it is important to clearly establish the *chief complaint(s)* that led the individual to seek help. The chief complaint(s) can be elicited through questions such as

"What brought you here?" "Tell me, what are your concerns?" "How can I be of help to you?" If the individual has more than one complaint, a list of the current problems is compiled in the interviewer's mind. As the interview progresses, the seven dimensions of each symptom or problem are explored.

In the exploration for cultural information, the clinician should pay particular attention to the sociocultural *setting* through which the illness experience is mediated. As Morgan and Engel have noted (12), whether it be a place the patient is in, an activity he or she is doing, or in a relationship with someone, the setting provides the context in which the symptom is experienced. The interviewer is alerted to opportunities to pursue the patient's own ideas about himself or herself, the patient's illness and the environment, and his or her relations to the symptoms or event. The individual's own beliefs on causation, the particular manner or idiom in which the symptoms are expressed, and the rituals or procedures taken to alleviate or exacerbate the symptoms or complaints are noted. When all of this information is considered together, a rich context for the life experience of the patient should emerge that provides a coherent cultural context for the patient's present conflicts and stresses. Cultural information elucidated in the interview can then be sorted out and organized according to the CF outline in Table 5–1. Cultural data are then integrated into the formulation of a diagnosis and treatment plan.

The following case illustrates the relevance of cultural materials and the application of the CF in psychiatric diagnosis and care.

Case Example

Present History

The patient is a 22-year-old graduate student of Korean American background who sought psychiatric consultation for the chief compliant of depression. He has difficulty concentrating on his schoolwork, and his grades are falling. He expresses feeling pain "like grieving or tearing something inside."

He feels angry with a lot of things and expresses intensification of his feeling of loneliness since his father was recently jailed in

Korea for political reasons. He has also recently broken up with his girlfriend.

The patient expresses ambivalent feelings toward his father. As a son, he cares a lot about his father. As an adult who now has strong Western political, religious, and social values reflective of his upbringing in the United States, he agrees that his father should be punished for his alleged wrongdoings.

The patient feels increasingly depressed, which he describes as emotional pain as he became increasingly aware of his feelings. He admitted to fleeting suicidal thoughts but has made no actual attempts because he feels a sense of obligation to those who count on him for support, particularly his siblings.

Past Psychiatric History

During his college years, the patient had a period of brief psychotherapy with a female Caucasian psychotherapist. The experience left him feeling "dehumanized" and "disempowered." Expecting the therapist to be more responsive to him, he interpreted the therapist's bodily gestures, passive demeanor, and unresponsiveness to him as "patronizing."

Past General Medical History

His general health has been good except for low back pain that worsens when he is tired or stressed.

Family History

The patient's father was in the military before entering politics. He was described as a disciplinarian and had been physically abusive to the patient. The patient's mother was described by him as having "obsessive-compulsive" traits as well as being "delusional and hysterical." Constant quarreling, angry outbursts, and bitterness mark the relationship between his parents. One of his two siblings has a depressive illness.

Personal History

Growing up in Korea, the patient felt isolated and abused and had few friends. Although he did fairly well academically, he never quite fit in among his peers. The family immigrated to the United States as political exiles and settled in the South for a few years before the parents moved back to Korea, leaving behind the patient and his siblings. During his high school years, he converted to Christianity. Christianity gave him, for the first time in his life, existential meaning and the collegial relationship among friends he had long sought.

The patient sees his identity as Korean American. He speaks English fluently and speaks little Korean. Even in the United States, he feels more like an exile and finds it difficult to relate to other Korean Americans. He considers himself to be a "left-wing Christian," imbued with the teaching of Jesus Christ to help the poor. He admires American values of openness, acceptance of a weak and vulnerable nature, tolerance, and freedom.

In contrast, the patient dislikes the hierarchical structure of Korean society. Although producing remarkable material advances, he considers the Korean culture controlling, violent, and promoting strong martial and patriarchal tendencies with a "no-questions-asked" environment. He feels that the Korean military mentality condones corporal punishment of children, and he blames the culture as promoting the physical abuse he experienced in his family.

After college, he decided to enter the ministry. When he learned that his father was imprisoned in Korea for political reasons, he became extremely stressed. With the added stresses of breaking up with his girlfriend, the pressure of schoolwork, and moving to a new environment, he became progressively more depressed. Suicidal thoughts of crashing his car crossed his mind but were never acted out. He sought therapy to change himself and to seek symptomatic relief.

Mental Status Examination

The patient is alert, oriented to time, person, and place. He maintains eye contact most of the time. He speaks in a soft manner with a deliberate pace. He has a good command of the English language. His vocabulary indicates that he is well educated. His thought processes are logical, sequential, and goal directed. Although his mood is depressed, he has no suicidal ideation. His insight is good and he is introspective. He is unsure of his future. He appears motivated to seek therapy.

Diagnostic Formulation

Axis I	296.23	Major depressive disorder, single episode, severe, without psychotic features
	V62.89	Religious or spiritual problem
Axis II		None
Axis III		Low back pain of unknown etiology
Axis IV		Degree of stress: severe
		Psychosocial stressors: father's imprisonment, breakup with girlfriend, mental illness of sibling, pressure of schoolwork, moving to a new city
Axis V		GAF: Past year 70
		Current 55

General Case Formulation

Biological. Genetic predisposition is suggested by the presence of probable mental illness in this patient's parents and sibling.

Developmental. The patient lacked emotional nurturance from his parents, who appeared incapable of providing the love and attention he needed. Such distancing of affect from his parents created in him a craving for love and attention. Repeated attempts at intimacy were rebuffed and reinforced with physical abuses. He developed tremendous anger toward his father, which is displaced to all authority figures.

Psychological. Dynamically speaking, the basic conflicts experienced by the patient are 1) independence versus dependence, 2) activity versus passivity, 3) adequate self-esteem versus diminished self-esteem, and 4) unresolved or delayed grief. These are reflective of the basic universal conflict situations James Mann mentioned (13). The conflict is expressed through an extreme ambivalence toward his parents, particularly his father, a craving for intimacy yet fear of making a commitment in any relationship, tardiness in therapy, hypercriticism of others, and a diffusion of his sense of identity.

Sociocultural.   Having been raised in a Korean culture with inculcation of a paramount respect for his elders, the patient experienced tremendous guilt feelings once he realized how angry he is with his parents. Because of his perceived social reinforcement of the Korean military culture, he rebels strongly against any authority figure. During his teenage years, he experienced a period of emotional upheaval when he exhibited problematic behavior in school.

His upbringing in the United States provided him with contrasting Western values of freedom, respect for the individual, and the nurturance he cherishes. The transformation of his personality occurred when he converted to Christianity. For the first time, he found meaning to his existence. He decided to become a minister.

Yet the unresolved anger, pain, grief, and unreconciled ambivalence remained. The imprisonment of his father brought to fuller consciousness his hatred toward his father. Blaming himself, albeit unconsciously, the patient plunged into a severe depression. He also began to question whether he was making a right choice in entering the ministry.

Course and Outcome

One-to-one, insight-oriented psychotherapy is prescribed to provide symptomatic relief and insight into his problem. Antidepressant therapy is withheld pending the results of psychotherapy. Spiritual counseling for his ambivalence toward the ministry is also recommended.

Cultural Formulation

The cultural context of the patient's illness experience, summarized below, conveys the cultural antecedents to the nature of his inner conflict as an individual that is reflected in the confusion and ambivalence about his identity. It also connects the psychosocial events to his recent depression. It further sheds light on the potential impact of his past relationships on the relationship with his current therapist.

1. *Cultural identity.* He assumes a dual identity, both Korean and American. Yet this identity is not solidified. He speaks primarily English with little Korean. He retains many traditional Korean cultural values, but his current values are primarily Western. He has not yet comfortably and fully integrated within himself both Korean and Western values. This diffusion of cultural identity creates ambivalence about himself, his relationship with his parents, and his career choice.

2. *Cultural explanations of the individual's illness.* The patient's predominant idioms of distress through which symptoms or the need for social support are communicated are shaped by the Western emotional concept and construct of illness. He has assimilated many Western values and beliefs. He is fairly in tune with a Freudian psychological construct of conflict, defenses, stresses, insight, conscious, and unconscious materials and the use of verbal therapy as a means of seeking relief from his distresses.

3. *Cultural factors related to psychosocial environment and levels of functioning.* His stresses stem primarily from an unresolved conflict, a feeling of extreme ambivalence toward his parents that he unconsciously displaces to all authority figures. He craves the intimacy he has not had and yet fears being rebuffed when he gets close to people. This is compounded by cultural factors in that he experienced his culture as reinforcing a sense of control over himself, which he rebels against. His religion has been a source of support to him, offering not only the circle

of friends he needed but providing him with an outlet for sublimating his anger by helping others through a commitment to social causes and to the ministry. The contrasting Eastern and Western cultural values and beliefs within him have been a source of conflict.

4. *Cultural elements of the relationship between the individual and the clinician.* Prior therapeutic experience with a Caucasian woman therapist has been disappointing to him in that he interpreted the therapist's more passive and neutral stance as unnurturing, unsupportive, and demeaning. This may be a transference problem in that the woman therapist had assumed the role of an "uncaring" mother. He needs a more nurturing and supportive type of clinician-patient interaction. His present relationship with an Asian male therapist appears to assuage his fear in that the present therapist, as compared with the previous female Caucasian therapist, is more understanding of his Asian culture. However, as therapy progresses, transference predictably will involve the feelings of ambivalence he has had toward his Asian father.

5. *Overall cultural assessment for diagnosis and care.* The patient clearly identifies with both the Korean and the North American cultures. Without a resolution of his ambivalence, the conflict can continue to play out in many situations and can interfere in his relationships and in his career. Individual psychotherapy is indicated to resolve this core conflict and depression. A male therapist who is familiar with both Asian and Western cultures would clearly be ideal for him. However, the ambivalence and negative transference of anger is to be anticipated as therapy progresses.

The prognosis is good. He has many areas of ego strength, is insightful, and is motivated to seek insight-oriented therapy at present.

Spiritual counseling, along with psychotherapy, would be useful to assist him in resolving his ambivalence toward his career choice as a minister.

Application of CF in this case puts the experience of the patient's illness in the context of the Korean American culture and not just the dominant U.S. Caucasian cultural background and avoids stereotyping. It brings out a clearer understanding of the psychological issues with which the patient is struggling. Therapeutic intervention is likewise tailored to meet his needs.

■ CONCLUSION

The sociocultural setting provides the *context* through which meanings about an individual illness are mediated (10). To elucidate cultural information, CF can be a useful guideline. In the elucidation of cultural information, it is essential for patients to sense that the interviewer is interested in such information and will not pass judgment. A biopsychosocial approach to health and disease provides the scientific framework to explore this heretofore neglected cultural area. Mastery of the associative interview equips the interviewer with the necessary tool to elucidate pertinent cultural data. Cultural information is best obtained during exploration in the course of a regular psychiatric interview using an associative technique of interviewing. Adding cultural context to the biopsychosocial approach to health and disease gives a fuller, unbiased understanding of an individual's illness experience and allows prescription of more appropriate therapies.

■ REFERENCES

1. Lewis-Fernandez R: Cultural formulation of psychiatric diagnosis. Cult Med Psychiatry 20:133–144, 1996
2. American Psychiatric Association: Diagnostic and Statistical Manual of Mental Illness, 4th Edition, Text Revision. Washington, DC, American Psychiatric Association, 2000
3. Lu FG, Lim RF, Mezzich JE: Issues in the assessment and diagnosis of culturally diverse individuals (American Psychi-

atric Press Review of Psychiatry, Vol 14). Edited by Oldham JM, Riba MB. Washington, DC, American Psychiatric Press, 1995, pp 477–510

4. Gaw AC (ed): Culture, Ethnicity and Mental Illness. Washington, DC, American Psychiatric Press, 1993

5. Mezzich JE, Kleinman A, Fabrega Jr H, et al (eds): Culture and Psychiatric Diagnosis. Washington, DC, American Psychiatric Press, 1996

6. Tseng WS, Streltzer J (eds): Culture and Psychopathology. New York, Brunner/Mazel, 1997

7. Engel GL: The clinical application of the biopsychosocial model. Am J Psychiatry 137:535–544, 1980

8. Engel GL: Psychological Development in Health and Disease. Philadelphia, PA, WB Saunders, 1964

9. Feinstein AR: Clinical Judgment. Baltimore, MD, Williams and Wilkins, 1967, pp 24–25

10. Kleinman A: Rethinking Psychiatry: From Cultural Category to Personal Experience. New York, Free Press, 1988

11. Bernstein RL, Gaw AC: A proposed classification of koro in the DSM-IV. Am J Psychiatry 147:1670–1674, 1990

12. Morgan ML, Engel GL: The Clinical Approach to the Patient. Philadelphia, PA, WB Saunders, 1969

13. Mann J: Time-Limited Psychotherapy. Cambridge, MA, Harvard University Press, 1973

6

CROSS-CULTURAL PSYCHOPHARMACOLOGY

Cross-cultural psychopharmacology, a relatively young field (1), is the special area of pharmacology that deals with the variations in psychotropic drug responses in different populations and the contribution of pharmacological factors to such variations (2).

In recent years, this field of study has grown as data have accumulated regarding variations in response to psychopharmacological treatment of psychiatric disorders across different ethnic and cultural groups. These data consist of 1) clinical and pharmacological investigations documenting different therapeutic dosage regimens in persons of different cultural background, and 2) discovery of pharmacogenetic polymorphisms in similar ethnic groups.

In the discussion of cross-cultural psychopharmacology, the terms *ethnicity, culture,* and *race* are often used interchangeably. Strictly speaking, *ethnicity* relates to "races or large groups of people classed according to common traits" (3). *Race* refers to "individuals grouped according to shared genetic characteristics" (3), whereas *culture* is defined as "sets of standards for behavior that govern human behavior" (4). Thus, race, ethnicity, and culture are similar in that they identify groups of people but are different in that this identity is determined either by phenotype, genotype, or shared customs or behavioral characteristics.

Steven K. Branch, M.D., Ph.D., contributed to this chapter and the preparation of tables.

In this chapter, I review the contribution of pharmacokinetic, pharmacogenetic, and pharmacodynamic factors to the variations of psychotropic drug responses in different populations.

■ OVERVIEW

A drug must be present in an appropriate amount at its loci of action to exert its desired effects. Both biological and environmental factors determine the concentration of a drug in various tissues. Biological factors include the amount of drug administered, extent and rate of its absorption, distribution, protein binding, localization in tissue, biotransformation, and excretion (5). The schematic pathways to drug effects are shown in Figure 6–1.

Other biological factors such as age, body size, fat content, general health status, gender, race, and the activity of genetically determined drug-metabolizing enzymes also influence the action of drugs (5). Environmental factors include diet, tobacco consumption, alcohol consumption, concomitant use of other nonpsychotropic medications, herbal medicines, food, and dietary products

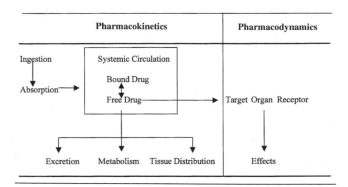

FIGURE 6–1. **Schematic presentation of the pharmacokinetic and pharmacodynamic pathways of drug effects.**
Source. Adapted from reference 6.

with varying protein and carbohydrate composition (5). Sociocultural factors include physicians' biases, patients' beliefs and expectations, placebo effects, and patient compliance (6). The study of the relationship of the dose of a drug and the utility of that drug in the treatment of human diseases is referred to as *pharmacokinetics* and *pharmacodynamics* (5). *Pharmacokinetics* refers to the general bodily response to the presence of xenobiotics (such as drugs) in the human body. It includes the biochemical and physiological processes involved in the process of absorption, distribution, metabolism (biotransformation), and excretion of a drug that determine the drug's final plasma concentration (5). *Pharmacodynamics* refers to biochemical and physiological effects of drugs at their loci of actions in the body (5). *Pharmacogenetics,* on the other hand, is the special area of biochemical genetics that deals with variation in drug response and the contribution of genetics to such variation. This field can broadly encompass any genetically determined variation in responses to drugs or, in a narrower sense, be restricted to those variations that are revealed only by response to drugs or other chemicals (2).

Culture as learned behavior is intimately related to biological processes. Although the metabolism of xenobiotic compounds is determined biologically, the selection and preferential use of various substances and drugs are learned behaviors and primarily culturally determined. Thus, the interrelationship of cultural and biological factors must be taken together in determining drug effects.

■ PHARMACOKINETICS

Metabolism or chemical biotransformation of drugs plays a prominent role in the pathway of a drug in the human body (Figure 6–1). The metabolism of xenobiotics leading to deactivation (although some drugs are prodrugs and require metabolism for conversion to the active form [e.g., codeine to morphine]) is accomplished by phase I or phase II reactions that render drugs more polar- and lipid-soluble before excretion, primarily through the kidneys (5). (Note that some drugs are prodrugs and require metabo-

lism for conversion to the active form [e.g., codeine to morphine].)
Phase I reactions involve the chemical process of oxidation, reduction, or hydrolysis typically by the cytochrome P450 enzyme (5). Examples of psychoactive medications that undergo phase I reactions are *N*- and *O*-dealkylation of desipramine, side-chain (aliphatic) and aromatic hydroxylation of phenobarbital and phenytoin, sulfoxide formation of chlorpromazine, deamination of amphetamine, and desulfuration of thiobarbital. *Phase II reactions* are conjugation reactions and involve the coupling of the drug or the polar metabolite with an endogenous substrate such as glucuronate, sulfate, acetate, or an amino acid. Glucuronidation of diazepam is an example (5).

P450 Enzyme

Cytochrome P450 plays a major role in the metabolism of both endogenous compounds, such as steroids, bile and fatty acids, prostaglandins, and biogenic amines, and exogenous compounds, such as drugs, carcinogens, pesticides, hydrocarbon, steroids, plant products, and pollutants (7). Likewise, hepatic P450 enzymes are found to be involved in the metabolism of psychotropic medications. P450 enzymes are classified in Figure 6–2, using 2D6 as an example.

Those proteins from all sources with a 40% or greater sequence identity are included in the same family and designated with an arabic number (e.g., 2). Those with greater than 55% identity

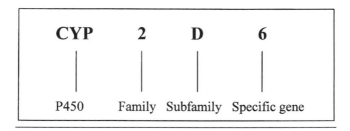

FIGURE 6–2. **Notation of the P450 enzyme CYP2D6.**

(>55% homology) are included in the same subfamily and designated by a capital letter (e.g., D). The individual genes and gene products are arbitrarily assigned arabic numbers (6).

Of the 16 cytochrome P450 enzymes currently identified in human tissues, only 7 are present in significant quantities in the liver: CYP1A1/2, 2A6, 2C9/10, 2C19, 2D6, 2E1, and 3A3/4/5.

Oxidative Reactions Catalyzed by Cytochrome P450

Hepatic cytochrome P450 isoenzymes, which are located at the smooth endoplasmic reticulum of the liver and catalyze the oxidative reaction in phase I metabolism of most drugs, are known as the *monooxygenases* (5). Embedded in the lipid bilayer of the smooth endoplasmic reticulum in the liver and in close proximity are two classes of P450 isoenzymes, *cytochrome hemoprotein* and *nicotinamide adenine dinucleotide phosphate–cytochrome reductase* (NADPH-cytochrome reductase). These two P450 enzymes, together with molecular oxygen, actively participate in the conversion of the xenobiotic substrates into oxidized products (Figure 6–3).

In the above oxidative reaction, the xenobiotic substrate (drug) first reacts with the oxidized (Fe^{3+}) cytochrome P450 to form an enzyme-substrate complex. The resulting drug-cytochrome complex accepts an electron contributed by NADPH through the NADPH-cytochrome P450 reductase to form a reduced complex. A molecule of oxygen plus a second electron and two hydrogen ions contributed by the same NADPH-flavoprotein-cytochrome P450 reductase then react with the reduced complex to form an activated oxygen intermediate product. Finally, an oxidized metabolite is formed with the transfer of an atom of oxygen to the substrate; a second atom of oxygen combines with free hydrogen to form H_2O. With the regeneration of the oxidized cytochrome P450, the oxidized iron molecule is ready for the next oxidative cycle (5).

Oxidized metabolites are mostly inactive and more water soluble than the original drug. However, some metabolites remain pharmacologically active, such as norfluoxetine from fluoxetine, and secondary amine tricyclic antidepressants (TCAs) from the ter-

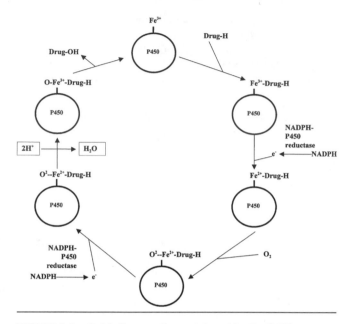

FIGURE 6–3. **Oxidative reaction catalyzed by the P450 enzymes.**
Source. Adapted from reference 5.

tiary amine TCAs. This accounts for the prolonged pharmacological action of fluoxetine.

Mechanisms Affecting P450 Enzymatic Activities

The rate of cytochrome P450 protein activity is influenced by substrates that either induce or inhibit its production.

Inducers increase the synthesis of P450 enzyme and have the effect of increasing the rate of biotransformation and reducing the serum level of the parent compound. Following are examples of substances that induce the synthesis of hepatic P450 enzyme:

- CYP1A: Polycyclic aromatic hydrocarbons from industrial pollutants, cigarette smoke, charbroiled meat, phenytoin, omeprazole, and *R*-Warfarin (8)
- CYP3A4: Glucocorticoids and anticonvulsants (phenobarbital, phenytoin, and carbamazepine), rifampin, and *R*-Warfarin (8)

Inhibitors decrease the synthesis of P450 enzymes and usually result from competition between two or more drugs for the active site of the same enzyme. The effects are an increased serum level of the less-metabolized parent compound, prolonged pharmacological effect, and increased incidences of drug-induced toxicities. Following are examples of inhibition that involve P450s:

- CYP1A2: Fluvoxamine, cimetidine, α-naphthoflavone, troleandomycin (8)
- CYP2D6: Quinidine, fluoxetine, norfluoxetine, paroxetine, sertraline, cimetidine, amiodarone (8)
- CYP3A4: Nefazodone, erythromycin, clarithromycin, troleandomycin, ketoconazole, itraconazole, fluconazole, astemizole, naringenin, gestodene (8)

Certain drugs such as secobarbital and ethinyl estradiol are referred to as *suicidal inactivators* because they form permanent complexes and render the P450 enzyme inactive (5).

Coadministration of the antifungal agent ketoconazole, the antihistamine astemizole, and terfenadine may result in an increased level of these drugs through inhibition of metabolism via CYP3A4 and may result in potential serious consequences including cardiac arrthymia of *torsades de pointes* and death (9). These drugs should never be coadministered. In addition, some drugs, including the antidepressant nefazodone, are also inhibitors of CYP3A4. Nefazodone should never be coadministered with terfenadine, astemizole, or cisapride. The concomitant use of nefazodone with other selective serotonin reuptake inhibitors (SSRIs) may result in competitive inhibition of CYP3A activity and should also be avoided.

Effects of Diet on Pharmacokinetics

Diet has been found to alter the pharmacokinetic reaction of drugs. It was shown that a steady diet consisting of charbroiled beef could reduce peak phenacetin plasma levels by 78% (10). A similar increase in antipyrine metabolism induced by dietary factors was also documented in Sudanese people living in Britain and Caucasian British residents versus Sudanese who remained in their country of birth (11). This was subsequently demonstrated to be caused by the induction (overexpression) of liver cytochrome P450 enzymes (12) as occurs with phenobarbital, antipyrine, or rifampin pretreatment (13), and smoking or exposure to cigarette smoke.

Grapefruit juice has been found to inhibit CYP1A2 and CYP3A4 (12). The active ingredient of grapefruit juice, 6′,7′-dihydroxybergamottin, is responsible for the inhibitory effect on CYP3A4.

A diet high in cruciferous vegetables such as cabbage, broccoli, and brussels sprouts has been found to reduce blood phenacetin levels by as much as 67% through inhibition of CYP1A2 by indole-3-carbinol, a chemical common to these vegetables (12). Thus, it is important to keep the patient's diet in mind as a potential confounding factor when evaluating drug effects.

Effect of Protein-Binding Transport on Pharmacokinetics

Although less well studied, ethnic variation has been reported in both the structure and the quantity of both α-1-C glycoprotein and albumins in human blood (8). These proteins are involved in the transport of drugs in the blood. Variation in plasma protein binding sites and quantity may be reflected in differential levels of plasma unbound drugs. Psychotropic drugs such as imipramine, chlorpromazine, fluphenazine, loxapine, thioridazine, thiothixene, carbamazepine, and triazolam have been shown to have a higher affinity for α-1-C glycoprotein than for albumin (14). Nortriptyline, amitriptyline, and methadone have been shown to increase binding affinity to an S (slow) variant of the α-1-C glycoprotein (14).

Interethnic difference has been shown in absolute levels of α-1-C glycoprotein as well as the distribution of its S (slow) and F (fast) variants (14). The frequency of the S variant in various populations ranges as follows: 54% among Indians from Mexico, 43%–45% among Canadian Eskimos and South American Indians, 34%–67% among African Americans and Caucasians in the United States and Europe, and 15%–27% among Orientals (14).

■ PHARMACOGENETICS

Polymorphism occurs when two or more alternative genotypes are present together in a population, each at a frequency greater than that which could be maintained by recurrent mutation alone and is reflected in a bimodal or trimodal distribution of the activity of a drug-metabolizing enzyme (2). Polymorphism may result in deficient or impaired enzymatic activities. The monogenic variation of cytochrome P450 enzymes expression results in a trimodal distribution of drug metabolism with classification of individuals within a group as either poor, intermediate, or extensive metabolizers (11, 15). *Poor metabolizers* (PMs) are those with enzyme mutation(s) resulting in deficient enzymatic activities. Those with a normal amount of enzyme are called *extensive metabolizers* (EMs). Those individuals with amounts of enzymes in between are *intermediate* or *slow metabolizers* (SMs). PM populations have been shown to have increased blood levels of drugs metabolized by the affected enzyme and also higher incidences of drug-induced side effects. For both historical interests and clinical reasons, the following clinical observations are noted regarding the discovery of genetic polymorphism among different ethnic groups.

Glucose-6-Phosphate Dehydrogenase Deficiency

Deficiency of glucose-6-phosphate dehydrogenase (G6PD), an X-linked enzyme, is estimated to affect 400 million people worldwide. G6PD deficiency is related to resistance to malarial infection. One allele, the variant, is found in 1 in 20 African American males

(2). Deficiency of G6PD was discovered when hemolytic anemia was induced in some patients after the antimalarial drug primaquine was given to African American male soldiers fighting in World War II.

Subsequently the mechanism of the hemolysis was clarified. The oxidized form of glutathione causes cell oxidative damage. A product of G6PD is NADPH (Figure 6–2). NADPH protects the cell against oxidative damage by regenerating reduced glutathione from the oxidized form. In D6PD deficiency, oxidant drugs such as primaquine deplete the cell of reduced glutathione. The consequent oxidative damage leads to hemolysis (2).

In parts of the Mediterranean where G6PD deficiency is prevalent, ingestion of fava beans is known to result in *favism,* a severe hemolytic anemia. G6PD deficiency is also a major cause of both neonatal jaundice and congenital nonspherocytic anemia (2).

Acetylation Polymorphism

When test doses of isoniazid, a drug used in the treatment of tuberculosis, were administered, the rate of disappearance of isoniazid from plasma showed a bimodal distribution in the population. This led to the identification of individuals as *rapid* or *slow acetylators.* Slow acetylators have a substantial decrease in the quantity of the arylamine N-acetyltransferase in the liver (16). About 5%–20% of Asians compared with 50% of African Americans and up to 65% of Caucasians are slow acetylators. Acetylation polymorphism has been implicated in the differential response between Asians and Caucasians to isoniazid toxicity: Asians are reported to have higher incidences of obstructive jaundice, whereas Caucasians have higher incidences of peripheral neuritis (17).

In addition to isoniazid inactivation, acetylation reactions are associated with the following clinical phenomena in rapid acetylators (16):

- A higher failure rate of weekly isoniazid therapy for tuberculosis
- Need for higher doses of hydralazine to control hypertension

- Need for larger doses of dapsone to treat leprosy and other infections

The following clinical phenomena are found in slow acetylators:

- Greater risk of developing drug-induced systemic lupus erythematosus–like syndrome while receiving hydralazine therapy
- Increased risk of developing hematological adverse drug reactions after isoniazid treatment
- Increased incidences of bladder cancer when exposed to carcinogenic arylamines (17)

Aldehyde Dehydrogenase Deficiency in Asians and Native Americans

Alcohol is first oxidized by the enzyme alcohol dehydrogenase (ADH), then acetaldehyde is further oxidized to acetic acid by the enzyme aldehyde dehydrogenase (ALDH). Toxic accumulation of plasma acetaldehyde, an intermediate product in the metabolic degradation of alcohol following alcohol consumption, produces the characteristic "flushing response." About 85%–90% of Asians are EMs with regard to ADH_2, a form of alcohol dehydrogenase (18). Furthermore, about 50% of Chinese and Japanese but not Malays are deficient in aldehyde dehydrogenase. For Asians who show the above genetic variations, there is a rapid conversion of alcohol to acetaldehyde but a slower degradation of acetaldehyde to acetic acid. This leads to a rapid accumulation of toxic plasma acetaldehyde that results in the characteristic symptoms of facial flushing as well as tachycardia, dysphoria, nausea, and vomiting (18).

■ CYTOCHROME P450 POLYMORPHISM

The drugs and the known enzymes responsible for their oxidation are summarized in Table 6–1. CYP2D6, CYP2C19, and possibly CYP2B6 and CYP1A2 are genetically polymorphic; that is, there are different forms of the same enzyme due to alterations in the genetic sequence. These mutations (six different variants have been documented for CYP2D6 alone) often result in a nonfunctional

TABLE 6–1. Comparison of poor metabolizers (PM) of psychotropic medications among U.S. Caucasians, Asian Americans, African Americans, and Hispanic Americans

Drug	Enzyme(s) involved in oxidation	% PM Caucasian	% PM Asian American	% PM African American	% PM Hispanic American
Antipsychotics					
Thioridazine	CYP2D6[a]	5%–10%	1%–2%	2%	4.5%
Perphenazine	CYP2D6	5%–10%	1%–2%	2%	4.5%
Thiothixene	?CYP3A4				
Haloperidol	?CYP3A4				
Clozapine	CYP1A2,[b] CYP2D6, FMO3				
Risperidone	CYP2D6	5%–10%	1%–2%	2%	4.5%
Olanzapine	CYP1A2				
Antidepressants					
Amitriptyline	CYP2C19,[c] CYP1A2, CYP2D6	2%–6%	20%	?	?
Doxepin	CYP1A2				
Imipramine	CYP2C19, CYP1A2, CYP2D6	2%–6%	20%	?	?
Protriptyline	CYP1A2				
Clomipramine	CYP2C19, CYP1A2, CYP2D6	2%–6%	20%	?	?
Fluoxetine	CYP2D6, others?	5%–10%	1%–2%	2%	4.5%
Sertraline	CYP2D6, CYP3A4[d]?	5%–10%	1%–2%	2%	4.5%
Paroxetine	CYP2D6, others?				
Fluvoxamine	CYP1A2, CYP2D6				
Venlafaxine	CYP2D6, CYP3A4	5%–10%	1%–2%	2%	4.5%
Bupropion	CYP2B6[e]	15%?	70%?	?	?
Nefazodone	CYP3A4, others?	5%–10%	1%–2%	2%	4.5%

Mood stabilizers				
Carbamazepine	CYP3A4		?	?
Anxiolytics				
Diazepam	CYP2C19	2%–6%	20%	?
Alprazolam	CYP3A4			
Midazolam	CYP3A4			
Triazolam	CYP3A4			

Note. % PM is included only for the first enzyme listed in the column. ? or blank = unknown or unreported data.

[a] CYP2D6 provides a classic example of genetic polymorphism; inhibited by some SSRIs, TCAs, and neuroleptics; also found in the brain.

[b] CYP1A2 may demonstrate genetic polymorphism; induced by cigarette smoke.

[c] CYP2C19 is inhibited by tranylcypromine, fluvoxamine, and fluoxetine; induced by rifampin; demonstrates genetic polymorphism.

[d] CYP3A4 is autoinducible.

[e] CYP2B6 has an unknown genetic polymorphism; induced by phenobarbital and carbamazepine.

Source. Data adapted from references 11, 12, 19, and Gaviria M, Gil A, Javid JI: "Nortriptyline Kinetics in Hispanic and Anglo Subjects." *Journal of Clinical Psychopharmacology* 6:227–231, 1986.

enzyme that leads to a subsequent increased drug response caused by failure to eliminate the drug (15). Additionally, there may be no response at all secondary to an inability to convert a prodrug to its metabolically active form, as in the case of the conversion of codeine to morphine by CYP2D6 (11, 15). Therapeutic failure has also been reported in patients who were classified as ultrarapid metabolizers (11, 15). There was an amplification of CYP2D6 that resulted in efficient elimination of specific target psychotropic compounds and an inability to achieve adequate serum drug levels. Duplication of CYP2D6 has been reported in 7% of a Spanish population (11).

Among all the P450 enzymes, polymorphism of two cytochrome P450 isoenzymes, CYP2D6 and CYP2C19, has been most extensively studied. CYP2D6 is responsible for the oxidative process in the metabolism of the following psychotropic medications:

- TCAs
- SSRIs
- Typical neuroleptics
- Atypical neuroleptics including clozapine and risperidone

The SSRIs (paroxetine, fluoxetine, norfluoxetine, and sertraline) are inhibitors of CYP2D6.

Table 6–1 provides PM rates for different populations. Although fewer Asians are PMs as compared with Caucasians, approximately one-third of Asians have been found to have gene mutations that significantly decrease the activities of CYP2D6 (19). The net result is CYP2D6 ratios of metabolic activity that are intermediate (SM) between those of EMs and PMs. This led to an overall lowered CYP2D6 activity in Asians compared with that in Caucasians (6).

Although the percentages of PMs among Caucasians listed in Table 6–1 are representative for Americans and Europeans, the data for African Americans do not adequately reflect the percentages found in Africans. In fact, there is wide variability between populations in different regions of Africa. With regard to CYP2D6, 2% of Zambians, 0%–7% Ghanaians, 0%–8% Nigerians, and 19% of San Bushmen from South Africa are PMs (11). Whether this reflects ethnic isolation secondary to limited extratribal marriages or is the result of environmental influences such as diet is unknown. There is evidence that diet not only induces enzyme upregulation (see above) but may also inhibit enzyme action (20).

CYP2C19 is involved in the metabolism of the following drugs:

- Diazepam
- Demethylation of tertiary TCAs (imipramine and amitriptyline)
- Citalopram
- SSRIs

SSRIs (fluoxetine, fluvoxamine, sertraline) are inhibitors of CYP2C19.

The molecular basis of the enzymatic defect in CYP2C19 in PMs recently has been reported (20) to be a single base pair mutation, G → A, in exon 5. This has an aberrant site that alters the reading frame to produce a protein lacking the heme-binding region and renders the enzyme nonfunctional (21).

■ ETHNIC VARIATIONS IN PHARMACOKINETICS OF PSYCHOTROPIC MEDICATIONS

As discussed earlier, pharmacokinetic parameters describe how the body handles xenobiotics and are a means of determining the metabolic phenotype coded for by the genes. In 1962, differences in mean daily doses between Europeans and North Americans (United States) of butyrylperazine and haloperidol were noted (22). Later, differences in haloperidol doses were noted even among British, French, and Swiss patients (23). Because these investigations involved Caucasian, eurocentric groups, differences in therapeutic levels could be attributed to culture, body morphology (percentage of body fat and redistribution of lipophilic compounds), age (decreased renal or hepatic clearance) (24), or even dietary differences.

Subsequent controlled studies indicated that haloperidol plasma levels were observed to be increased, sometimes as much as 50% in Asian patients with schizophrenia, as compared with Caucasians in several studies even after controlling for body surface area differences. Additionally, durations of peak plasma levels of haloperidol were shorter for Asians, reflecting slower metabolism of this compound. This was true for both Asians residing in their homeland and immigrants to the United States, which indicates that environmental factors were less of an influence than genetics. In keeping with these observations, the major metabolite of haloperidol was found to be increased in the serum of Asians (25, 26). If CYP3A4 is indeed the cytochrome P450 enzyme responsible for the metabolism of haloperidol, the above observations suggest that the enzyme CYP3A4 demonstrates genetic polymorphism. No information is currently available for pharmacokinetics of haloperidol in African Americans; however, studies with both trifluoperazine and fluphenazine revealed no ethnic difference in any of the parameters (27). No pharmacokinetic studies are currently available for the Hispanic population (28).

Table 6–2 presents plasma half-life, rate of clearance, and time to peak plasma levels for various psychotropic drugs in different ethnic populations. Among the TCAs, desipramine and nortriptyline clearances in Asians were significantly lower than those in Caucasians. In keeping with a reduced rate of clearance, desipramine peak plasma time was also considerably shorter (1, 25). Although the cytochrome P450 enzymes responsible for the metabolism of desipramine and nortriptyline have not been identified, the reduced pharmacokinetic parameters of these drugs suggest that CYP2C19 may be involved. Not only is this enzyme less prevalent in Asian populations, it has also been documented to oxidize other TCAs. African American patients treated with either nortriptyline or amitriptyline had 50% higher plasma levels of nortriptyline than did Caucasians (29); however, no significant increase was observed with amitriptyline. In a study of patients who had overdosed with TCAs, plasma concentrations were greater in African Americans than in Caucasians (27). These studies suggest that two different enzymes may be responsible for the metabolism of nortriptyline and amitriptyline and that a significant degree of genetic polymorphism may be discovered among African Ameri-

TABLE 6–2. Comparison of pharmacokinetic parameters of psychotropic medications among major U.S. ethnic minority groups

Drug	Caucasian			Asian			African American			Hispanic		
	$t_{1/2}$	CL	T_{max}	$t_{1/2}$	CL	T_{max}	$t_{1/2}$	CL	T_{max}	$t_{1/2}$	CL	T_{max}
Antipsychotics												
Haloperidol (25)	14.1–18.8	33–49	NA	NA	NA	NA	NA	NA	NA	NA	NA	NA
Fluphenazine[a]	14.8	NA	NA	NA	NA	NA	11.5	NA	NA	NA	NA	NA
Trifluoperazine[b]	12.9	607.4	2.50	NA	NA	NA	18.9	638.1	2.96	NA	NA	NA
Antidepressants												
Nortriptyline[c]	26.5	32 (6.7[d])	7.8	NA	32	NA	NA	NA	NA	27.6	6.7[d]	9.4
Desipramine	NA	178[d]	414	NA	1.27[d]	240	NA	NA	NA	NA	NA	NA
Mood stabilizers												
Lithium (26)	15.9	NA	NA	14.1	NA	NA	20.9	NA	NA	NA	NA	NA
Anxiolytics												
Alprazolam (29)	12.6	3.91	44.4	15.8	3.05	44.4	NA	NA	NA	NA	NA	NA
Adinazolam (30)	7.11	62.4	1.81	6.44	37.8	2.59	6.1	49.2	3.1	NA	NA	NA

Note. Values reported from p.o. administration. $t_{1/2}$ = half-life (hours); CL = clearance (L/hour); T_{max} = peak plasma time (minutes); NA = not available.

[a]Data from Midha KK, Hawes EM, Hubbard JW, et al.: "Variation in the Single Dose Pharmacokinetics of Fluphenazine in Psychiatric Patients." *Psychopharmacology (Berlin)* 96:206–211, 1988.

[b]Data from Midha KK, Hawes EM, Hubbard JW, et al.: "A Pharmacokinetic Study of Trifluoperazine in Two Ethnic Populations." *Psychopharmacology (Berlin)* 95:333–338, 1988.

[c]Data from Gavira M, Gil A, Javaid JI: "Nortriptyline Kinetics in Hispanic and Anglo Subjects." *Journal of Clinical Psychopharmacology* 6:227–231, 1986.

[d]in L/kg·hour.

cans. In Hispanics, nortriptyline pharmacokinetic parameters are similar to those of Caucasians (28).

A slower clearance rate for diazepam was observed in Asian subjects; however, subsequent studies failed to bear out that observation, especially after data was corrected for body fat percentages (25). When the anxiolytics alprazolam and adinazolam were investigated, Asians showed lower half-lives and clearance of the drugs as compared with Caucasians even after body fat corrections were made. African Americans demonstrated pharmacokinetic parameters for adinazolam that were intermediate with respect to Caucasians and Asians (30, 31). As in studies of ethnic population treated with haloperidol, these data suggest that CYP3A4 is genetically polymorphic. What is unusual is that in subsequent studies, diazepam was not shown to have significantly different pharmacokinetics in Asians as compared with Caucasians, despite being metabolized by a cytochrome P450 enzyme known to display considerable pharmacogenetic variability. This suggests that another enzyme is involved in diazepam oxidation. Additionally, environmental factors may be more significant with regard to the metabolism of diazepam, and thus the Gaussian distribution seen under these conditions (15) may mask typical Mendelian (monogenic) influences.

Of special note are the pharmacokinetics of lithium. No differences are observed for kinetic parameters between Asians and Caucasians; however, in African Americans lithium has a longer half-life and a significantly higher red blood cell/plasma ratio. This is partially due to reduced efficiency in the lithium-sodium countertransport protein in African Americans. Red blood cell lithium levels are believed to correlate with neuronal levels, and suggested lithium dosage requirements may need to be lowered for African Americans (27, 31).

■ PHARMACODYNAMICS

Pharmacodynamics describe the effect a drug has upon the body, both beneficial effects and side effects (1). Table 6–3 presents ther-

TABLE 6-3. **Comparison of therapeutic dosages of antipsychotic and antidepressant medications among major U.S. ethnic minority groups**

Drug	Caucasian	Asian	African American	Hispanic
Antipsychotics				
Haloperidol (25)	10	6.5 (24)	NA	NA
Clozapine	450	NA	NA	300 (27)
Risperidone	4–8	NA	NA	6 (27)
Chlorpromazine	400, 599 (32)	347 (34), 258 (32)	NA	397 (32)
Antidepressants				
Amitriptyline	150	169 (34)	NA	NA

Note. Therapeutic doses are reported as maintenance dose (mg/day). References are included in parentheses. NA = not available.

apeutic dosage values as reported in the literature for various populations as well as the occurrence of side effects. In addition to differences in recommended therapeutic amounts of psychotropic medications, psychodynamic parameters can be evaluated with the occurrence of side effects. In a study examining chlorpromazine usage in Caucasians, Asians, and Hispanics, movement disorders were documented in significant numbers of Asians and Hispanics as compared with Caucasians despite the use of lower therapeutic doses (32). Asians on a fixed dose of haloperidol, which was in the therapeutic range for Caucasians, also had more extrapyramidal symptoms as compared with a control group (25).

Asians also respond favorably to the treatment of depression with imipramine and desipramine at lower doses and have a lower threshold for side effects (1). In one study, Hispanic women used only approximately half the dose of TCAs and complained more frequently of side effects than did Caucasian women (1). What role cultural influences play in the interpretation of this data is unknown. African Americans treated with imipramine demonstrated more rapid improvement than did Caucasians (33). Additionally, African Americans treated with TCAs were more likely to develop delirium, as were older patients (33).

In contrast with the lack of lithium pharmacokinetic differences in Asians and Caucasians, therapeutic levels are documented to be lower: 0.5 to 0.8 meq/L in Asians and 0.8 to 1.2 meq/L in Caucasians (25). Lithium dosages in African Americans, which are similar to those for Caucasians, are associated with a greater frequency of reported side effects (34), which is in keeping with a slower half-life and possible greater intraneuronal lithium concentration.

In the past decade, the allele frequencies for polymorphisms at several loci of interest to neuropsychiatry have been determined in samples of individuals from different populations. Loci that have been proposed to be associated with psychiatric illnesses are listed in Table 6–4.

In one study, blood samples were drawn from the following populations: European (Adygei), Native Americans (Maya of the

TABLE 6–4. **Polymorphisms at loci of neuropsychiatric interest and their proposed relation to psychiatric illness**

Locus	Psychiatric disorder
Tryptophan hydroxylase (TPH)	Suicide-related behaviors and impulsivity
Dopamine transporter protein (SLC6A3)	Susceptibility to cocaine-induced paranoia and attention-deficit disorder
D3 dopamine receptor (DRD3)	Schizophrenia and bipolar affective disorder
Ciliary neurotrophic factor (CNTF)	Psychosis
μ-Opioid receptor (OPRM1)	Substance dependence
Apolipoprotein E	Alzheimer's disease

Source. Adapted from reference 35.

Yucatan and Rondonia Surui from the Amazon basin), Australo-melanesian (Nasioi), sub-Saharan African (Mbuti Pygmies), and East Asian (Chinese). Significant allele frequency variation among populations was found at all six loci listed in Table 6–4 (35).

Although the functional significance of susceptibility to various psychiatric disorders and behavioral phenomena must await further studies, Gelernter et al. (35) pointed out that knowledge regarding polymorphisms of receptor genes at loci of neuropsychiatric interest can be important to elucidate genetic variation in receptor foci. Designs for such studies should include research subjects recruited from different population groups.

■ CONCLUSION

Recent advances have revealed significant differences in the metabolism of psychotropic drugs among various cultural/ethnic populations; these differences affect the treatment of psychiatric disorders. Considerations of pharmacogenetic, pharmacokinetic, and pharmacodynamic parameters in drug therapy will allow for optimization of dose and avoidance of side effects. This is especially significant in light of an increasing minority population in the United States and the shift of population pattern in the world. Although current methodologies into genotypal/phenotypal characteristics of individuals are limited to research settings, data from these investigations have helped us begin to establish guidelines for appropriate therapy. Clinicians are advised to take these factors into consideration when prescribing psychotropic medications.

■ REFERENCES

1. Sramek JJ, Pi EH: Ethnicity and antidepressant response. Mt Sinai J Med 63:320–325, 1996

2. Thompson MW, McInnes RR, Willard HF: Genetics in Medicine, 5th Edition. Philadelphia, PA, WB Saunders, 1991

3. Kalow W: Ethnic differences in drug metabolism. Clin Pharmacokinet 7:373–400, 1982

4. Goodenough WH: Comments on cultural evolution. Daedalus 90:521–528, 1961

5. Benet LZ, Kroetz DL, Sheiner LB: Pharmacokinetics: the dynamic of drug absorption, distribution and elimination, in Goodman and Gilman's The Pharmacological Basis of Therapeutics, 9th Edition. Edited by Hardman JG, Limbird LE. New York, McGraw-Hill, 1996

6. Lin KM, Poland RE: Ethnicity, culture, and psychopharmacology, in Psychopharmacology: The Fourth Generation of Progress. Edited by Bloom FE, Kupfer DJ. New York, Raven, 1995, pp 1907–1917

7. Coon M, Ding X, Pernecky S, et al: Cytochrome P450: progress and predictions. FASEB J 6:669–673, 1992

8. Shen WW: Cytochrome P450 monooxygenases and interactions of psychotropic drugs: a five year update. Int J Psychiatry Med 25:277–290, 1995

9. Woolsey RL, Chen Y, Freiman JP, et al: Mechanism of the cardiotoxic actions of terfenadine. JAMA 269:1532–1536, 1993

10. Conney AH, Pantuck EJ, Hsiao KC, et al: Enhanced phenacetin metabolism in human subjects fed charcoal-broiled beef. Clin Pharmacol Ther 20:633–642, 1976

11. Edeki T: Clinical importance of genetic polymorphism of drug oxidation. Mt Sinai J Med 63:291–300, 1996

12. Jefferson JW: Drug interactions—friend or foe? J Clin Psychiatry 59 (suppl 4):37–47, 1998

13. Eichelbaum M: Polymorphic drug oxidation in humans. Federation Proceedings 43:2293–2302, 1984

14. Mendoza R, Smith MW, Poland RE, et al: Ethnic psychopharmacology: the Hispanic and Native American perspective. Psychopharmacol Bull 27:449–461, 1991

15. Kalow W: Pharmacogenetics in biological perspective. Pharmacol Rev 49:369–379, 1997

16. Grant DM, Morike K, Eichelbaum M, et al: Acetylation pharmacokinetics. J Clin Invest 85:968–972, 1990

17. Weber WW: The Acetylator Genes and Drug Responses. New York, Oxford University Press, 1987

18. Goedde HW, Agarwal D (eds): Alcoholism: Biomedical and Genetic Aspects. New York, Pergamon, 1989

19. Smith MW, Mendoza RP: Ethnicity and pharmacogenetics. Mt Sinai J Med 63:285–290, 1996

20. de Morias SM, Wilkinson GR, Blaisdell J, et al: The major genetic defect responsible for the polymorphism of S-mephenytoin metabolism in humans. J Biol Chem 269:15419–15422, 1994

21. Lewis P, Rack PH, Vaddadi KS, Allen JJ: Ethnic differences in drug response. Postgrad Med J 56 (suppl 1):46–49, 1980

22. Chrusciel TL: Questions we recognize but cannot formulate. International Pharmacopsychiatry 13:112–117, 1978

23. Kinirons MT, Crome P: Clinical pharmacokinetic considerations in the elderly: an update. Clin Pharmacokinet 33:302–312, 1997

24. Lin, KM, Poland RE, Smith MW, et al: Pharmacokinetic and other related factors affecting psychotropic responses in Asians. Psychopharmacol Bull 27:427–439, 1991

25. Froemming JS, Lam YWF, Jann MW, et al: Pharmacokinetics of haloperidol. Clin Pharmacokinet 17:396–423, 1989

26. Strickland TL, Ranganath V, Lin KM et al: Psychopharmacologic considerations in the treatment of black American populations. Psychopharmacol Bull 27:441–448, 1991

27. Ramirez LF: Ethnicity and psychopharmacology in Latin America. Mt Sinai J Med 63:330–331, 1996

28. Ziegler VE, Biggs JT: Tricyclic plasma levels: effect of age, race, sex, and smoking. JAMA 238:2167–2199, 1977

29. Lin, KM, Lau JK, Smith R, et al: Comparison of alprazolam plasma levels in normal Asian and Caucasian male volunteers. Psychopharmacology (Berl) 96:365–369, 1988

30. Ajir K, Smith M, Lin KM et al: The pharmacokinetics and pharmacodynamics of adinazolam: multi-ethnic comparisons. Psychopharmacology (Berl) 129:265–270, 1997

31. Lawson WB: The art and science of the psychopharmacotherapy of African Americans. Mt Sinai J Med 63:301–305, 1996

32. Strickland TL, Stein R, Lin KM: The Pharmacologic treatment of anxiety and depression in African Americans: considerations for the general practitioner. Arch Fam Med 6:371–375, 1997

33. Flockhart DA: Drug interactions and the cytochrome P450 System. Clin Pharmacokinet 29 (suppl 1):45–52, 1995

34. Rosenblatt R, Tang SW: Do oriental psychiatric patients receive different dosages of psychotropic medication when compared with occidentals? Can J Psychiatry 32:270–273, 1987

35. Gelernter J, Kranzler H, Lacobelle J: Population studies of polymorphisms at loci of neuropsychiatric interest (tryptophan hydroxylase [TPH], dopamine transporter protein [SLC6A3], D3 dopamine receptor [DRD3], apoliproprotein E [APOE], μ opioid receptor [OPRM1], and ciliary neurotrophic factor [CNTF]). Genomics 52:289–297, 1998

7

CULTURAL CONTEXT OF NONADHERENCE TO PSYCHOTROPIC MEDICATIONS IN PSYCHIATRIC PATIENTS

Nonadherence, defined as "the extent to which the patient's behavior (in terms of taking medications, following diets, or executing other lifestyle changes) *does not* coincide with medical or health advice [emphasis added]" (1), is a widespread and serious challenge in the United States. Sackett and Haynes (2) estimate that at least 50% of patients do not adhere to physicians' prescribed medication regimens. In various cultural settings, psychotropic medication nonadherence is a serious and prevalent problem among psychiatric patients. A follow-up study (3) of 406 patients 2 years after discharge from a psychiatric hospital in South Africa revealed nonadherence rates for oral phenothiazines of two-thirds for black patients, one-half for colored patients, and one-quarter for white patients. Kelly and Scott (4) estimate that between 35% and 65% of outpatients with schizophrenia and other chronic psychotic conditions do not adhere to prescribed medications. Van Putten (5) found that approximately 31% of patients with bipolar disorder did not take prescribed lithium and/or stopped coming to the treatment facility. Kinzie and colleagues found that, despite given adequate

John A. Nichols, Psy.D., contributed to the research and writing of this chapter.

tricyclic antidepressant (TCA) dosages, 61% of the refugee patients treated for depression with TCAs at their Indochinese clinic showed no TCA level in their blood. Another 24% revealed very low serum TCA levels. Close to 50% of psychiatric patients refuse medications at some time during their treatment (6). Clearly, non-adherence to psychotropic medications is a serious challenge. The association of drug nonadherence with high relapse rates highlights the importance of aggressively addressing this issue in clinical practice (7).

A comprehensive literature review of all factors associated with nonadherence to medications in various populations is beyond the scope of this chapter. However, in this chapter I first provide an overview of some key factors that affect nonadherence to psychotropics medications in psychiatric patients. I then focus on those sociocultural factors that affect psychopharmacotherapy and the issue of nonadherence. Next I introduce and propose the use of an instrument that I and John A. Nichols have developed, Clinician's Inquiry Into the Meaning of Taking Psychotropic Medications (currently unpublished), as a tool in assessing nonadherence to psychotropic medications in clinical practice. Finally, I summarize some practical measures to enhance medication adherence.

■ OVERVIEW OF FACTORS IN PSYCHOTROPIC DRUG NONADHERENCE

Table 7–1 lists some of the important factors to consider when encountering drug nonadherence in a psychiatric patient. The clinical questions linked to each factor in the table can be used as a guide in the differential diagnosis of the problem of psychotropic medication nonadherence.

Drug Side Effects

Concern about side effects is almost invariably present in a patient receiving psychotropic medications. Often, a patient's complaints of uncomfortable side effects (e.g., antipsychotic drug effect on

TABLE 7–1. **Differential diagnoses of medication nonadherence in psychiatric patients**

Side effects and effects of drugs

Are side effects contributing to nonadherence?

Is the diagnosis correct?

Are the right drugs being prescribed?

Are the dosages of drugs correct?

Is the best route of administration of drug given?

Is there drug-drug interaction?

Are there other substances, dietary products, and environmental products interfering with drugs' action?

Education: Is there sufficient education provided for the patient?

Drug effects and side effects

How to take drugs

How to judge improvements and approximately when to expect improvement

How long to take medications

What to do if side effects/emergency occur

How to make changes of medications

What food, medications, or other substances to avoid while on medications

Health beliefs: Is there any incongruity between the patient's beliefs and prescriber's notions of health beliefs on drugs?

What does it mean for the patient to take medications?

Why do the medications work or don't work for the patient now?

What would happen if drugs were continued?

Does the size, color, and form of medications have any adverse meanings?

Psychodynamics

Is there a significant lack of insight by the patient pertaining to psychotherapy and treatment (especially treatment with medication)?

Are the defense mechanisms of projection, denial, identification, or displacement interfering with medication adherence?

Is medication seen as symbolic in any of the following ways: as a transitional object, as poison, as being sexualized, as reinforcing the "sick" label?

Is medication consult symbolic of a secret, illicit, or forbidden meaning?

Transference

Is the patient's transference involved with medication refusal?

(continued)

TABLE 7–1. **Differential diagnoses of medication nonadherence in psychiatric patients (*continued*)**

Countertransference
    Are there potentially detrimental countertransference reactions (e.g., anger and/or distancing)?

Anger
    Is the patient's anger and/or acting out of aggression interfering with medication adherence?

Psychosis
    Is psychosis possibly contributing to medication nonadherence in ways such as capriciousness, delusional thinking, or hypomania?

Cognition
    Are cognitive difficulties such as poor memory interfering with taking medications?

Relationship factors
    Is the clinician fostering a collaborative relationship with the patient?

Sociocultural factors: What sociocultural factors may be involved in actual or potential medication nonadherence?
    Is family support present?
    Are there family members who would influence patient in taking medication?
    Are there significant others who may influence patient in taking medication?
    Does the patient subscribe to alternative system of healing?
    Is the patient taking herbal drugs?
    Are there religious beliefs against taking of medications?

thinking, sedative effect of antidepressants, and long-term side effects of tardive dyskinesia) and medications not achieving their desired effects may lead to a patient discontinuing his or her medications. Real concern about the side effects of a drug is further compounded by increasing findings concerning the influence of variations in gene structure on drug metabolizing capacity among various ethnic and racial groups (see Chapter 6, Cross-Cultural Psychopharmacology).

While it is critical to attend to the physiological differences in drug metabolism and drug-induced side effects, and to correctly prescribe drugs for accurately diagnosed clinical problems, it is also important to be cognizant of the meaning of side effects in patients' experiences. Patients' attributed meanings to side effects often contribute to nonadherence. For example, side effects involving sexual function can be a particularly alarming experience. For certain individuals, this is a significant threat to their "virility" or "femininity" and self-esteem. Other patients may be concerned about carcinogenic effects or other catastrophic physical and/or mental effects if they take psychotropic drugs. It behooves the clinician to understand and query this complex and often emotionally laden view of side effects. Interventions can then be tailored to the particular concerns of the patient.

Knowledge

Frank (8) suggested that knowledge deficits, not only on the part of the patient but also on the part of the prescribing clinician, are relevant to treatment adherence. Salzman (9) noted a positive correlation between knowledge and psychopathology and its treatment when treating the elderly population. The use of psychoeducational technique has been advocated as a significant tool in fostering medication adherence.

Health Beliefs

The patient's own explanatory models and beliefs of psychopathologies and treatment modalities, including ideas of effective drugs, are important factors to consider when assessing drug nonadherence (10, 11). Incongruity between the patient's beliefs and prescriber's notions of health beliefs concerning drugs has been found to lead to nonadherence (12). It behooves the clinician to carefully elicit the patient's own beliefs about psychopathologies and drug effects when assessing a potential or actual nonadherence problem. This is especially important for certain ethnic and immigrant groups. For example, clinicians who have treated Asian Americans and Hispanic Americans have often heard the concerns from such groups that Western medicines are too strong and have more side effects than do herbal drugs (6, 10). Such complaints should be taken into consideration and the basis of the patient's beliefs explored in order to make effective interventions.

The symbolism of drugs and potential patients' reactions to them may be another factor to consider relating to nonadherence. Perceptual characteristics of size, form, and color of drugs were found to vary with ethnic group with regard to expected drug effect (12). In a study comparing the perceptual characteristics of size, form, and color of drugs and their expected effects between black and white undergraduate psychology students, appreciable differences were noted for size-strength relationship and drug action expectancies with colors of capsules. In general, white subjects seemed more color oriented in forming expectations of drug actions. They also preferred capsules over tablets (12). The comparative meanings of colors of drugs and drug expectation are summarized in Table 7–2.

Reasons for the comparative differences in color-associated expectations of drug effects and the pervasive effect of this influence on drug nonadherence are unclear. Although cultural factors are suspected, differences in age, socioeconomic status, and drug experience cannot be ruled out. Nonetheless, it is important to keep this possibility in mind.

Psychodynamics

Many authors have noted the relevance of psychodynamics when dealing with the patient who does not adhere to medication. For example, Book (13) highlighted the defense mechanisms of projection, denial, identification, and displacement believed to be used by nonadherent patients. Furthermore, medication could be viewed as a transitional object, symbolically allowing an ongoing continuous relationship with a protective figure, even when seeing the psychiatrist infrequently. This variation of nonadherence can take the form of the patient *not* wanting to discontinue a medication (13).

TABLE 7–2. **Comparative meanings of colors of drugs and expected drug effects between white and black undergraduate students**

Color of drug	Black subjects	White subjects
White capsule	Stimulants	Analgesics
Black capsule	None	Stimulants, analgesics
Orange capsule	Weak stimulants	Stimulants
Yellow capsule	Psychedelics	Stimulants
Light green capsule	Sedatives	None

Source. Adapted from reference 12.

Transference

One of the more dramatic components of the clinician-patient encounter, and how it relates to drug taking, has to do with the mobilization of transference reactions. This factor in nonadherence is particularly evident in patients with borderline personality disorder. Waldinger and Frank (14) stated that patients with borderline personality frequently experience profound, dramatic, and unstable transference reactions to the prescribing clinicians and to the medication itself. These shifting intrapsychic and interpersonal dramas often negatively affect the treatment. For example, prescribing medications may foster regressive trends in individuals with borderline personality, increase control struggles, and trigger other complicated emotionally charged states (14). Thus, clinicians should note the salient difficulties when treating a patient with borderline personality disorder. As Brockman (15) has noted, "Without an understanding of the reciprocal potential of medication and transference, one is left very much in the hands of the patient to evaluate results, to assess side effects, and potentially at the mercy of the patient's regressive wish to maintain control and overcome fear by sacrificing the goals of the treatment for the sake of these regressive needs" (p. 294). The impact of transference as it relates to medication compliance is still an understudied area.

Clinician's Countertransference

Just as it is important to note the saliency of the patient's transference, the significance of the clinician's own countertransference (reaction to patients stemming from the experience of the clinician's own background) has been noted in the experience of dealing with a patient who is not adhering to medication (16, 17). Hostility within the clinician is a distinct possibility and could foster antitherapeutic behaviors reflected in prescribing medication. Conscious or unconscious hostility toward patients may lead to their early discharge or under- or overmedication. Thus, these emotional states within the prescribing clinician, as well as those in the patient, are germane in the management of the issues involved.

Clinician-Patient Relationship

A realistically based therapeutic alliance between the patient and the clinician is important in the implementation of treatment plans, including medication. Listening to the patient, increasing staff contact, increasing availability to the prescribing clinicians, and forming long-term relationships are important factors not only in fostering drug adherence but also in dealing with concerns about medication effects. As Appelbaum and Guthiel (18) have noted, "A closely supervised drug regimen in the context of a gratifying relationship with a skilled clinician is the most widely accepted prophylactic measure" (p. 341).

Anger and Psychosis

Anger and psychotic symptoms also may be factors in medication nonadherence. Van Putten and colleagues (19) found that the psychotic degree of ego-syntonic grandiosity, and reluctance by a patient to change this condition, is a powerful factor in drug refusal in individuals with schizophrenia. Some patients stop taking lithium because they do not want to lose the feeling of increased energy and creativity that is associated with "hypomania." The presence of delusion and fear of being poisoned is also a phenomenon frequently encountered with patients diagnosed with paranoid disorder. In addition, medication nonadherence has been seen as a convenient locus for the playing out of hostile and aggressive dynamics (20).

Cognitive Deficit

Salzman (21) noted that drug nonadherence in elderly patients is a significant problem. He observed that memory deficit and other cognitive difficulties, as well as physical limitations, are notable contributing factors.

Sociocultural Factors

Nonpharmacological factors in drug reactions and in nonadherence are also significant issues that are frequently neglected in both practice and research (10). This topic is further elaborated on below.

■ SOCIOCULTURAL FACTORS AFFECTING PSYCHOPHARMACOTHERAPY AND NONADHERENCE

Physicians prescribing medications and drug researchers interested in the efficacy of medication effects have long noted the importance of nonpharmacological factors such as the placebo effect in patients' responses to medications (10). These supposedly nonbiological effects, thought to be mediated through a symbolic mechanism, are estimated to range from 30% to 70% of the therapeutic responses with any treatment method (10). Yet, in spite of this, Lin and colleagues (10) noted that, paradoxically, in the midst of the current fervor of pharmacological research, less is known about and less research is directed toward the sociocultural and symbolic factors that affect drug responses than is directed toward the biological mechanisms mediated through kinetics, genetics, and dynamics (see Chapter 6, Cross-Cultural Psychopharmacology). What meager data we have are unsystematic and mostly anecdotal. In spite of this, it is important to begin addressing these nonpharmacological variables in drug responses. Some of the factors, such as health beliefs and nonadherence, have already been introduced and are further elaborated here. The following are some of the key sociocultural factors that are pertinent to the issues of psychopharmacotherapy and drug nonadherence:

1. Physician's biases in diagnosis and prescribing
2. Health beliefs
3. Concomitant usage of herbal and Western medicine
4. Diet
5. Placebo effect
6. Religious beliefs
7. The quantity and quality of social support (10)

Physician's Biases in Diagnosis and Prescribing

Physician's biases in prescribing are reflected in reports of racial differences in psychiatric diagnosis and psychotropic drug responses for many diagnostic categories. For example, although the U.S. Epidemiologic Catchment Area (ECA) study revealed no significant differences in the prevalence of affective disorders between African Americans and Caucasians (22), African Americans are more likely than Caucasians to receive a diagnosis of schizophrenia instead of affective disorder in clinical practice (23). A number of anxiety disorders, including obsessive-compulsive disorder, panic disorder, phobic disorder, and posttraumatic stress disorder, are often underrecognized or underdiagnosed in African Americans compared with Caucasians (24). The reasons for misdiagnosis remain unclear. However, the consequences of misdiagnosis for African American patients are the delayed implementation of appropriate medications such as lithium therapy for bipolar disorder, the prescribing of antipsychotic medications when not indicated, the use of higher dosages of antipsychotic medication and more frequent use of prn (*pro re nata*) medications, and the greater likelihood of receiving a depot medication (24).

Similarly, Hispanics with a confirmed diagnosis of bipolar disorder were far more likely to receive an initial diagnosis of schizophrenia (25). Heterogeneity among the Hispanic subgroups and the presence of culture-bound syndromes may also confound the diagnostic picture (26). Furthermore, some studies suggest that the dosage requirement for TCAs among Hispanic women may be different than for their Caucasian counterparts. A retrospective chart review of Hispanic female clinic patients showed a comparable treatment outcome when given only half the usual TCA dosage (27). Thus, if customary dosage of TCAs for Caucasians are prescribed for this population, the possibility of more complaints of side effects may occur. Indeed, Hispanic patients in this cohort were found to experience more side effects (78% vs. 33% for Caucasian patients) and to prematurely discontinue their medication (27).

Among Asian patients, failure to factor in body size and potential variance due to poor metabolizing enzymes may lead to greater incidences of side effects to psychotropic medications when these patients are given the usual recommended dosages.

Thus, some studies suggest that, among U.S. ethnic patients, drug dosages, patterns of drug usage, and drug nonadherence may differ from those of mainstream middle-class Caucasian patients (see Chapter 6, Cross-Cultural Psychopharmacology). Clinicians who are increasingly involved in the care of ethnic patients need to be cognizant of such variations in drug reactions.

Health Beliefs and Alternative Healing Traditions and Practices

In many non-Western cultures, a long tradition of an indigenous system of healing coexists with the modern Western scientific medical healing system. Examples of indigenous healing systems are the traditional Chinese medical system and Asian Indian Ayurvedic medicine. These traditional medical practices may influence patients' choices and reactions to modern treatment modalities, including drugs. For example, Chinese medical concepts, such as *chi's* and "energy flows," often shape the conceptions and responses of Chinese patients in the use of Western medicine (28). Indeed, discordance between professional and lay conceptions of causal attributions may determine a patient's satisfaction with treatment, medication adherence, and clinical outcome (10).

A study by Sing Lee (29) in Hong Kong is instructive and illustrates that patients' reactions to side effects of medications may vary according to their health beliefs. In a biocultural study of the report of side effects in 70 Hong Kong Chinese bipolar patients on chronic lithium therapy, Sing Lee found that there was an imperfect correspondence between biomedically founded and culturally endorsed psychotropic side effects. Contrary to the usual reports of Western patients, the Hong Kong patients did not usually regard polydipsia and polyuria as bothersome symptoms or translate them into metaphors to express undesirable side effects. Although complaints of tiredness, drowsiness, and poor memory were common, their frequency was significantly lower than in normal control subjects (Chinese subjects without a diagnosis of bipolar illness). Chinese patients had no conceptual equivalent to the complaint of "loss of creativity." Complaints of "missing of highs," loss of assertiveness, and fear of weight gain were rarely encountered (29).

When the author probed specifically for indigenous health beliefs in a nonjudgmental fashion, many patients were able to freely discuss their own indigenous notions of drug reaction. Thirty-eight percent of patients considered lithium to cause mild "hotness" that was readily neutralized by the "cooling effect" of water. The need for more water intake was not generally perceived to be an adverse symptom or side effect (polydipsia); rather, it was perceived to have a salutary effect. This conception stems from the idea of balancing "hotness" with "coolness" derived from traditional Chinese medicine. Similarly, drugs that were ascribed with properties of either "hotness," "coldness," or "dispersiveness" (a term describing general discomfort by dispersing the effects of drugs to other parts of the body) reflect this conceptual formulation based on yin and yang forces in the body (28). Therapeutic efforts were aimed as restoring any perceived yin/yang imbalance.

Health beliefs are often reflected in the varying ethnic expectations of Western and herbal drug actions. Many ethnic patients regard Western medications as providing quicker action and for treatment of acute illness (10). In contrast, some patients regard herbal drugs as having fewer tendencies to induce side effects (10) and delay or avoid taking necessary Western medications. Concerns about the addictive and toxic effects of drugs among U.S. Hispanics may lead them to avoid taking needed medications for longer periods and may lead to premature termination of medications and psychiatric care (10). On the other hand, in many Asian countries where the concoction of multiple herbal drugs in traditional medical practice is usually prescribed, polypharmacy may come to be an accepted norm of medical practice (10).

Thus, as noted earlier, drug-induced side effects often conjure up various intrinsic meanings for patients. Meanings such as feeling of being "less of a man" due to reduced potency or libido, feeling of being a "less useful member of society" due to decreased productivity, and increased dependency as when being restricted from driving due to the sedative effect of drugs may be significant unspoken reasons for drug nonadherence. To effectively address the issue of drug nonadherence, clinicians should pay attention to these explanatory models of drug action and effects to fully understand the patients' concerns.

Concomitant Use of Herbal and Western Medications

With the increasing popularity of the use of alternative healing methods in Western countries, the use of herbal drugs has also increased (30). More patients are now resorting to concomitant usage of herbal drugs and Western medicines. In the United States, this is especially true in some minority communities (10). Some herbal drugs have been shown to possess active pharmacological properties that may interact with current psychotropic medications (10). Some Chinese herbal drugs were found to induce P450 hepatic enzymatic actions (31) (Table 7–3).

Other herbs have an inhibitory effect. For example, through an inhibition of P450 that acts on their metabolites, oleanolic acid–containing Chinese medicinal plants such as *Sertia mileensis* and *ligustrum lucidium*, and schizandrin, corynoline, *Kopsia,* and clausenamide, were found to offer some hepatoprotective effects

TABLE 7-3. Induction effects of some Chinese medical herbs on P450 enzymes

Compound	Action	Clinical usage	Subjects
Schizandrin B, C Schizandrol B (tonic)	Induction	Hepatoprotective vs. viral hepatitis and drug-induced hepatitis	Rats
Corydalis bungeane Diels (herb)	Induction	Treatment of hepatitis	Mice
Kopsia officinalis lansium (herb)	Induction	Treatment of inflammation	Mice
Clausena lansium (fruit tree)	Induction	Treatment of viral hepatitis	Mice
Muscone (musk glands of male musk deer)	Induction	Increased clearance of pentobarbital, decreased pentobarbital-induced sleeping time	Rats
Ginseng (tonic)	Induction	Decreased pentobarbital-induced sleeping time	Mice
Glycyrrhiza (herb)	Induction	Reduced drug toxicity of various traditional Chinese medicines, reduced pentobarbital-induced sleeping time	Mice

Source. Adapted from reference 32.

against CCL_4-induced and acetaminophen-induced liver injury (31). Other herbal drugs such as the Japanese herb *Swertia japonica* have anticholinergic effect (10). These herbal drugs may interact with psychotropic medications and can confound the interpretation of drug effects and side effects. The effects of herbal drugs on psychotropic medications have generally not been well studied. More research is needed to elucidate herbal drug effects and their interactive effects with current psychotropic medications.

Diet

That different cultural groups have varying food preferences is a widely accepted fact. In recent years, there have been more studies that document the effect of diet on liver microsomal enzymes and the drugs metabolized by these enzymes. Cross-cultural differences of diet on metabolizing enzymes have been ably documented in a study comparing differences in biotransformation of drugs between Asian Indians living in India and those who have immigrated to Great Britain (31). The half-life of the rate of biotransformation of both antipyrine and clomipramine were shown to be longer for Asian Indians maintained on their traditional vegetarian diet as compared with those who had switched to a British diet (31, 32).

The average peak concentration of phenacetin, an analgesic, decreased by 78% when normal volunteers who were taking phenacetin were fed a charcoal-broiled diet for 4 days. This finding has been attributed to induction of the hepatic enzyme CYP1A2 involved in the metabolism of phenacetin (33).

Table 7–4 shows the enzymatic action of some commonly ingested fruit juices and cruciferous vegetables.

Grapefruit juice contains a furanocoumarin compound known as 6',7'-dihydroxybergamottin (34) that significantly inhibits CYP1A2 and CYP3A4, which leads to an increase in blood levels of drugs such as caffeine, cyclosporine, midazolam, triazolam, terfenadine, ethinyl estradiol, and a number of calcium channel blockers (35).

Cruciferous vegetables (broccoli, cabbage, brussels sprouts) contain a common chemical, indole-3-carbinol, that inhibits induc-

TABLE 7–4.	**Food products and their actions on P450 enzymes**	
Food	**Action**	**Enzymes**
Charcoal-broiled beef	Induction	CYP1A2
Grapefruit juice	Inhibition	CYP1A2, CYP3A4
Broccoli	Induction	CYP1A2
Cabbage	Induction	CYP1A2
Brussels sprouts	Induction	CYP1A2
Caffeine	Induction	CYP1A2
Ethanol	Induction	CYP2E1

Source. Adapted from Jefferson JW: "Drug Interactions: Friend or Foe?" *Journal of Clinical Psychiatry* 59 (suppl 4):37–47, 1998.

tion of CYP1A2. A reduction of blood phenacetin levels by as much as 67% have been shown in individuals on a diet rich in cruciferous vegetables (35).

Religious Beliefs

Certain religious groups discourage their members from taking medications. Patients with such strong religious beliefs who present with psychiatric symptoms such as uncontrollable bipolar mood swings may feel extremely conflicted and guilty when asked to take mood regulators. The chance of avoiding or discontinuing medications is high in such patients, and special efforts are needed to address their religious concerns and beliefs.

Placebo Effects

The placebo effect is presumably mediated through a symbolic mechanism and is estimated to account for 30%–70% of the therapeutic responses of any treatment (10). When the responses to the tricyclic trazodone and the antidepressant imipramine were compared for a matched groups of patients with endogenous depression consisting of Caucasians and African Americans in the United

States and Columbia, no significant differences were found between trazodone and placebo at any of the three groups. Imipramine was significantly better than placebo in all three groups, and the Columbian patients improved more regardless of treatment, including the placebo treatment (36). Thus, ethnic variation even in placebo effect should be kept in mind when assessing drug responses.

Quantity and Quality of Social Support

The quality and quantity of social support have been linked to treatment outcome and drug responses. Depending on the quality of family involvement, patients with high expressed emotion (EE) (characterized by frequent criticism, hostility, and emotional over-involvement) family members were found to be more likely to relapse on standard neuroleptic dosages (37, 38). Although limited, some data (39, 40) reveal that various ethnic groups vary with regard to their EE ratings. Some studies showed Caucasian American families more likely to have higher EE scores compared with their British counterparts. Hispanic families tend to have lower EE scores than do Caucasians in the United States and Britain (39, 40). Whether these findings translate into true causative factors for certain mental illnesses remains to be seen. Clinically, it is not difficult to appreciate the fact that when family members subject mentally ill patients to frequent negative criticisms, the patients will experience more stress and be more at risk to relapse despite adequate neuroleptic doses. Indeed, Liebermann and Strauss have shown that when bipolar patients were subjected to intense interpersonal conflicts, they experienced more relapses despite adequate lithium treatment (41).

On the other hand, the findings from two multinational follow-up studies on the outcome of schizophrenia by the World Health Organization (42) reveal a more favorable outcome in non-Western patients and note that these patients have more social support as compared with their Western counterparts. These findings lend credence to the postulate that social support influences the course of mental illness and the degree of adherence to psychotropic medications.

■ STRATEGIES FOR ENHANCING MEDICATION ADHERENCE

Keeping the above-mentioned factors affecting nonadherence in mind, we have developed a clinical protocol, *Clinician's Inquiry Into the Meaning of Taking Psychotropic Medications* (Table 7–5). This tool can be integrated into the interview when exploring a

---

TABLE 7–5.   Clinician's Inquiry Into the Meaning of Taking Psychotropic Medications

---

1. Do you have any feelings about taking medication(s)? What does it mean for you to take medication(s)?

2. What would your family, friends, or significant others think of you if you take medication(s)?

3. What, if any, are your concerns about the effects and/or side effects of your medication(s)?

4. Do you have any religious beliefs regarding the taking of medications?

5. What are the benefits of taking medications?

6. What are the benefits of not taking medications?

7. Would the color, size, or form of medications mean anything to you?

8. Do you have any concerns about losing control if you take medication? If yes, please elaborate.

9. Does the possibility of change, even if it is positive change, make you worried or uncomfortable? If yes, please elaborate.

10. Would taking medication change the way you view yourself? If yes, please elaborate.

11. Would taking medication affect your self-esteem? If yes, please elaborate.

12. Can you tell me more about your specific worries or dilemmas you have when thinking about medication?

---

patient's potential reaction to medications or when nonadherence emerges. Once the reason for nonadherence is identified, therapeutic strategies can be directed appropriately.

In addition, many authors have recommended various ways of enhancing patient's adherence to prescribed medications:

1. "Improving patients' levels of information concerning the specifics of their regimens, reinforcing essential points with review, discussion, and written instruction, and emphasizing the importance of the therapeutic plan" (43)
2. "Taking clinically appropriate steps to reduce the cost, complexity, duration, and amount of behavioral change required by the regimen and tailoring treatment regimens to suit the convenience of the patients" (43), such as prescribing once- or twice-daily dosing instead of three or four times daily, when clinically justifiable
3. Taking a health beliefs and drug-adherence history (43)
4. Improving the clinician-patient relationship and the patient's satisfaction with treatment (43)
5. Setting clear objectives of treatment goals and creating incentives for the patient's achievements (43)
6. Arranging for continuity of clinicians (43)
7. Involving the patient's family and support groups (43)
8. Enlisting assistance of all available health care workers, directed at improving adherence to treatment and medications (43)
9. Using depot medications (43)
10. Scheduling appointments before the patient's release from inpatient treatment (44)
11. Shortening the waiting period for an appointment (44)
12. Using prompts in the form of letters and telephone calls to encourage the patients to keep appointments (44)
13. Offering orientation and education about treatment and medications (44)
14. Aggressively treating of comorbid conditions such as substance use disorders (45)
15. Monitoring serum level of drugs (6)

16. Using ethnic-oriented clinics and matching ethnic patients with culturally competent therapists and prescribers (46)

■ CONCLUSION

Nonadherence to psychotropic medications in diverse populations remains a significant detriment to successful therapeutic outcome and involves complex and complicated variables. Nonadherence should be as seriously considered as other clinical issues when encountered during the treatment process. Taking a good history of patterns of drug use and of adherence or nonadherence to drug regimens in the first clinical interview and monitoring the issue throughout treatment can aid in anticipation of potential nonadherence problems. The patient's own explanatory model of drug effects needs to be elicited. Identifying and intervening in nonadherence is an integral part of drug prescribing, and reasons for nonadherence should be vigorously pursued. Carefully attending to, and working with, the variables of nonadherence increases the chances of a stronger clinician-patient relationship, better adherence, and a more successful outcome. More research into factors of nonadherence, including sociocultural variables, is needed.

■ REFERENCES

1. Haynes RB, Taylor DW, Sackett DL (eds): Compliance in Health Care. Baltimore, MD, Johns Hopkins University Press, 1979

2. Sackett DL, Haynes RB (eds): Compliance With Therapeutic Regimens. Baltimore, MD, Johns Hopkins University Press, 1976

3. Gillis LS, Trollip D, Jakoet A, et al: Non-compliance with psychotropic medications. S Afr Med J 72:602–606, 1987

4. Kelly GR, Scott JE: Medication compliance and health education among outpatients with chronic mental disorders. Med Care 28:1181–1197, 1990

5. Van Putten T: Why do patients with manic-depressive illness stop taking their lithium? Compr Psychiatry 16:179–183, 1975

6. Kinzie JD, Leung P, Boehnlein J, et al: Tricyclic antidepressant plasma levels in Indochinese refugees: clinical implication. J Nerv Ment Dis 175:480–485, 1987

7. Davis MS: Predicting non-compliant behavior. J Health Soc Behav 8:265–271, 1967

8. Frank E: Enhancing patient outcome: treatment adherence. J Clin Psychiatry 58 (suppl 1):11–14, 1997

9. Salzman C: Medication compliance in the elderly. J Clin Psychiatry 58 (suppl):18–22, 1995

10. Lin K-M, Poland RE, Nakasaki G (eds): Psychopharmacology and Psychobiology of Ethnicity. Washington, DC, American Psychiatric Press, 1993

11. Kleinman A: Rethinking Psychiatry. New York, Free Press, 1988

12. Buckalew LW, Coffield KE: Drug expectations associated with perceptual characteristics: ethnic factors. Percept Mot Skills 55:915–918, 1982

13. Book HE: Some psychodynamics on non-compliance. Can J Psychiatry 32:115–117, 1987

14. Waldinger RJ, Frank AF: Transference and the vicissitudes of medication use by borderline patients. Psychiatry 52:416–427, 1989

15. Brockman R: Medication and the transference in psychoanalytically oriented psychotherapy of the borderline patients. Psychiatr Clin North Am 13:287–295, 1990

16. Guthiel T: The psychology of psychopharmacology. Bull Menninger Clin 46:321–330, 1982

17. Guthiel T: Drug therapy: alliance and compliance. Psychosomatics 19:219–225, 1978

18. Appelbaum P, Guthiel T: Drug refusal: a study of psychiatric in-patients. Am J Psychiatry 137:340–346, 1980

19. Van Putten T, Crumpton F, Yale C: Drug refusal in schizophrenia and the wish to be crazy. Arch Gen Psychiatry 33:1443–1446, 1976

20. Raskin A: A comparison of acceptors and resistors of drug treatment as an adjunct to psychotherapy. J Consult Clin Psychology 25:366, 1961

21. Salzman C: Medication compliance in the elderly. J Clin Psychiatry 56 (suppl 1):18–22, 1995

22. Rob LN, Locke B, Regier DA: An overview of psychiatric disorders in America, in Psychiatric Disorders in America: The Epidemiologic Catchment Area Study. Edited by Robins LN, Regiers DA. New York, Free Press, 1991, pp 328–366

23. Adebimpe VR: Race, racism, and epidemiologic surveys. Hospital and Community Psychiatry 45(1):27–31, 1994

24. Lawson BL: Clinical issues in the pharmacotherapy of African-Americans. Psychopharmacol Bull 32:275–281, 1996

25. Murkerjee S, Shukla S, Woodline J: Misdiagnosis of schizophrenia in bipolar patients: a multi-ethnic comparison. Am J Psychiatry 140:1571–1574, 1983

26. Mendoza R, Smith MW, Poland RE, et al: Ethnic psychopharmacology: the Hispanic and Native American perspective. Psychopharmacol Bull 27:449–461, 1991

27. Marcos LR, Cancro R: Pharmacotherapy of Hispanic depressed patients: clinical observations. Am J Psychother 36:505–513, 1982

28. Gaw AC (ed): Culture, Ethnicity and Mental Illness. Washington, DC, American Psychiatric Press, 1993

29. Lee S: Side effects of chronic lithium therapy in Hong Kong Chinese: an ethnopsychiatric perspective. Cult Med Psychiatry 17:301–320, 1993

30. Eisenberg DM, Kessler RC, Foster C, et al: Unconventional medicine in the United States: prevalence, costs, and patterns of use. N Engl J Med 328(4):246–52, 1993

31. Allen JJ, Rack PH, Vaddadi KS: Differences in the effects of clomipramine on English and Asian volunteers: preliminary report on a pilot study. Postgrad Med J 53 (suppl 4):79–86, 1977

32. Liu G-T: Effects of some compounds isolated from Chinese medicinal herbs on hepatic microsomal cytochrome P-450 and

their potential biological consequences. Drug Metab Rev 23 (3–4):439–465, 1991

33. Fraser HS, Mucklow JC, Bulpitt CJ, et al: Environmental factors affecting antipyrine metabolism in London factory and office workers. Br J Clin Pharmacol 7:237–243, 1979

34. Edwards DJ, Bellevue FH, Woster PM: Identification of 6'7'-dihydroxybergamottin, a cytochrome P450 inhibitor, in grapefruit juice. Drug Metab Dispos 24:1287–1290, 1996

35. Jefferson JW, Greist JH: Brussel sprouts and psychopharmacology: understanding the cytochrome P450 enzyme system, in Psychiatric Clinics of North America: Annual of Drug Therapy. Edited by Jefferson JW, Greist JH. Philadelphia, PA, Saunders, 1996

36. Escobar JI, Tuason VB: Antidepressant agents: a cross-cultural study. Psychopharmacol Bull 16:49–52, 1980

37. Anderson CM, Reiss DJ, Hogarty GE (eds): Schizophrenia and the Family: A Practitioner's Guide to Psychoeducation and Management. New York, Guilford, 1986

38. Falloon IRH, Boyd JL, McGill CW (eds): Family Care of Schizophrenia: A Problem-Solving Approach to the Treatment of Mental Illness. New York, Guilford, 1984

39. Jenkins JH, Karno M: The meaning of expressed emotion: theoretical issues raised by cross-cultural research. Am J Psychiatry 149:9–12, 1992

40. Keefe SE, Padilla AM, Carlos ML: Emotional Support Systems in Two Cultures: A Comparison of Mexican Americans and Anglo Americans. Los Angeles, CA, University of California, Spanish Speaking Mental Health Center, 1978

41. Lieberman PB, Strauss JS: The recurrence of mania: environmental factors and medical treatment. Am J Psychiatry 141:77–80, 1984

42. Jablensky A, Sartorius N, Ernberg G, et al: Schizophrenia: manifestations, incidence and course in different cultures: a World Health Organization ten-country study. Psychol Med Monogr Suppl 20:1–97, 1992

43. Becker MH, Maiman LA: Strategies for enhancing patient compliance. J Community Health 6:113–135, 1980
44. Chen A: Noncompliance in community psychiatry: a review of clinical interventions. Hospital and Community Psychiatry 42:282–286, 1991
45. Keck PE, McElroy SL, Strakowski SM, et al: Compliance with maintenance treatment in bipolar disorder. Psychopharmacol Bull 33:87–91, 1997
46. Flaskerud J, Hu L-T: Participation in and outcome of treatment for major depression among low income Asian-Americans. Psychiatry Res 53:289–300, 1994

8

CULTURAL CONTEXT OF PSYCHOTHERAPY

Psychotherapists treating patients from diverse ethnic backgrounds not only face the challenge of bridging the linguistic and cultural gaps between their patients and themselves, but such cross-cultural encounters also may force psychotherapists to confront their basic assumptions about psychotherapy (1, 2). Consider the following six encounters within the cultural context suggested by Wohl (1):

1. An anthropologist or anthropologically oriented Western-trained psychiatrist or psychological clinician conducting research on the therapeutic modes and healing practices of another culture.
2. A Caucasian, middle-class, male therapist from a U.S. majority cultural group providing psychotherapy to an African American female patient, a member of a minority group in the United States.
3. A non-German speaking Cambodian refugee in Germany requiring psychotherapeutic intervention for an adjustment problem related to the host culture.
4. A visiting Western-trained psychotherapist in Thailand providing short-term psychotherapy to Thai patients.
5. A Chinese patient receiving Morita therapy in Japan.

6. The wife of an American businessman treated for depression through psychotherapy by a Chinese psychiatrist in Beijing, China.

These examples highlight the many logical possibilities in the vicissitudes of the meanings and techniques of the intercultural encounter. For example, what are the deeply held values, beliefs, and concepts of therapists that drive their therapeutic procedures? What are the moral and ethical positions regarding optimal outcome of psychotherapy for ethnic clients? Is Western-style psychotherapy applicable in all cultures? How does one reconcile a Western-based psychotherapeutic technique with indigenous helping strategies such as those derived from the Latino, Native, African, or Asian groups in the United States? How should psychotherapy be conducted within the context of a multicultural and ethnically diverse society? Are there universal variables common to all psychotherapies? How does the changing context in the current health care environment affect the patient-therapist relationship?

There are many forms and practices of psychotherapy, ranging from the insight-oriented dynamic Freudian approach to cognitive-oriented therapy. It is beyond the scope of this chapter to delve into these extant psychotherapeutic theories and practices. Rather, in the pages that follow, I first explore various psychotherapeutic issues when a therapist from one culture is called upon to provide psychotherapy to a patient from another culture. I then summarize therapeutic features common to all forms of psychotherapy. Furthermore, because an effective therapeutic relationship is essential for all therapeutic encounters, I examine how broad, macrosocial cultural variables affect both the process and structure of the therapist-patient relationship. Finally, in an attempt to bridge the conceptual gap between sociocultural and microphysiological variables, I adopt Kleinman's "sociosomatic" framework of analysis to indicate how such a conceptual map can serve to help us arrive at a biocultural theory of illness and healing. Underlying these discussions is the assumption that Western-style psychotherapy as is currently constructed and practiced needs to take into consideration the context of the local culture in order to have a more universal appeal and applicability in non-Western societies.

■ WHAT IS PSYCHOTHERAPY?

Broadly applied, *psychotherapy* refers to "verbal and nonverbal communications with patients as distinct from therapies that use, for example, drugs, surgery, or shock" (3). Within these parameters, psychotherapy "comprehends numerous kinds of activity believed to be therapeutic, among them suggestion, persuasion, hypnosis, catharsis, abreaction, identification, transference, psychodrama, group pressure, acting out, depth analysis involving the uncovering of unconscious materials through free association and dream interpretation, and education leading to the creation of insight" (4, p. 78). For purposes of discussion, I adopt the narrower definition provided by Frank, who defined psychotherapy as "a planned, emotionally charged, confiding interaction between a trained, socially sanctioned healer and a sufferer" (5). The terms *psychotherapy* and *counseling, cross-cultural* and *intercultural,* and *patient* and *client* are used interchangeably in this chapter.

Psychotherapy as a Cultural Phenomenon

Many authors have written about the inseparability of the practice of psychotherapy from its sociocultural context (1–7). Insofar that "culture is a great storehouse of ready-made solutions to problems which human animals are wont to encounter" (8, p. 54), psychotherapy itself, as part of a product of Western culture, probably has its parallels in every human society (1). "The therapeutic value of confession, be it to an individual or to a surrogate for the supernatural, is widely known to the clergy and the healing profession" (9). According to La Barre (9), "for a long time, psychiatrists have known the therapeutic value in one's simple, unfettered talking to another about his guilt and worries" (p. 36).

Because psychotherapists seek to interpret and transform the meanings of patients' communications, Frank concludes that psychotherapy resembles rhetoric and hermeneutics:

All psychotherapeutic endeavors, whatever their form, transpire entirely in the realm of meanings. All psychotherapies depend on the fact that human thinking, feeling, and behavior are guided largely by the person's assumptions about reality, that is meanings that he or she attributes to events and experiences, rather than their objective properties. (6)

Because culture provides the context in which the "reality" of a person's experience is perceived and interpreted, the study and application of the process and structure of psychotherapy cannot be divorced from its cultural context.

Common Themes in Intercultural Encounters in the Process of Psychotherapy

Kluckholn and Murray (8), in their classic book on personality and culture, reminded us that "every person in different ways is like all persons, like some persons, and like no other person." In other words, each person has characteristics that are universal, group-specific, and unique (10). Thus even though patients' backgrounds may vary, there still are some common themes frequently encountered when psychotherapy is transacted between a therapist and a patient of different cultural backgrounds (11):

1. *"The emic-etic distinction"* (11, p. 1): *what is culturally unique and universal in the counseling process? Emic* refers to what is unique within a local culture, whereas *etic* refers to the universal elements common to all human beings. In other words, the issue at hand is whether the task of therapy should be framed from the patient's emic perspective or that of the etic perspective of the therapist. Historically, there appears to be a tendency to believe that human distress is the same regardless of context and site and that the techniques to counteract it are effective everywhere. In fact, for a while among psychotherapists in the Boston area, there appeared a commonly held belief advanced by a well-known psychoanalyst that because human beings share similar emotions, the task of psychotherapy as

applied to all patients is the same, regardless of their cultural background. More recent studies have debunked this belief (1–7). It is now more commonly believed that cultural issues not only influence the psychotherapeutic process, but that the understanding and appropriate application of cultural principles is crucial in ensuring the acceptance of therapy by culturally diverse patients (5, 12).

2. *"The autoplastic-alloplastic dilemma"* (11, p. 8): *what are the goals of psychotherapy?* Whether the goal of therapy is to change oneself to accommodate the external circumstances (autoplastic) or to effect changes in the external environment (alloplastic) to relieve stress is highlighted by concerns over how goals should be set for patients who come from different cultural backgrounds with differing values. In the process of freeing individuals from psychological conflicts and of restructuring social situations that have brought the individual to therapy in the first place, should the end point in therapy be the patient's emancipation and liberation from his or her social context? Should therapists foster identity formation that is harmonious with patients' indigenous values or in conformity to that of the dominant society? What should the stance of therapists be when counseling international students or members of oppressed minority groups in the struggle against the oppressive nature of the social environment?

3. *"Relationship versus technique: what stays constant and what changes in cross-cultural counseling?"* (11, p. 10) It is generally assumed that regardless of the technical details of what is said in therapy, the importance of maintaining a therapeutic relationship is essential for effective psychotherapy (5). Thus, the therapist's acceptance of, respect for, and maintenance of ethical conduct toward patients remain immutable. Within this context, the general level of activity, mode of verbal or nonverbal communication, content of remarks, and tone of voice can be adapted to fit the unique needs of the patients at a particular time.

■ THE PROCESS OF PSYCHOTHERAPY: UNIVERSAL OR CULTURE SPECIFIC?

Various authors have raised the issue of whether Western-style psychotherapy is applicable to non-Western cultures (1, 2). Proponents of the universal approach, citing the robust Western-based counseling theories and techniques containing sufficient and necessary ingredients, believe psychotherapy should be effective with any patient, regardless of ethnicity (13).

Proponents of the culture-specific approach, on the other hand, argue for inclusion of culture-sensitive techniques unique to the patient's culture in order to meet the patient's specific needs (13). They argue that the inclusion of concepts, values, beliefs, and procedures of problem-solving that are congruent with the patient's culture make psychotherapy more effective (13).

Whether Western-style psychotherapy is universally applicable depends critically on the therapeutic features common to all forms of psychotherapy.

■ THERAPEUTIC FEATURES COMMON TO ALL TYPES OF PSYCHOTHERAPY

Much has been written about the therapeutic elements of psychotherapy and whether one technique is superior to another (5). Suffice it to say, the last words on the comparative efficacy of various types of psychotherapy are not yet in. Frank's works, nonetheless, summarized evidence of therapeutic features common to all types of psychotherapy as follows:

1. Patients who receive any form of psychotherapy do somewhat better than controls observed over the same period of time who have received no formal psychotherapy, which does not, of course, exclude their having benefited from informal helping contacts with others.
2. Follow-up studies seem to show consistently that whatever the form of therapy, most patients who show initial improvement maintain it.

3. More of the determinants of therapeutic success lie in the personal qualities of and the interaction between patient and therapist than in the particular therapeutic method used.
4. There are a few conditions in which the therapeutic method does make a significant difference in outcome. Behavior therapies seem to work better for phobias, compulsion, obesity and sexual problems than less focused therapies. Cognitive therapy seems particularly effective with depressed patients. (5, p. 15)

Frank concluded, "the efficacy of all procedures depends on the establishment of a good therapeutic relationship between the patient and the therapist. No method works in the absence of this relationship" (5, p. 15).

■ HOW DOES PSYCHOTHERAPY WORK?

Frank advanced a *demoralization hypothesis* that posits patients, whatever their symptoms, must share a type of distress that responds to the components common to all schools of psychotherapy: "Patients seek not for relief of symptoms alone, but for symptoms coupled with demoralization, a state of mind characterized by one or more of the following: subjective incompetence, loss of self-esteem, alienation, hopelessness (feeling that no one can help), or helplessness (feeling that other people could help but will not)" (5, p. 16). Demoralization is thought to manifest itself through subjective symptoms (anxiety, depression, loneliness) or behavioral disturbance (interpersonal conflicts). Frank suggests that improvement from psychotherapy lies in its ability to restore the patient's morale, with the resulting diminution or disappearance of symptoms (5). He posits the following four shared therapeutic components of all forms of psychotherapy as means directly or indirectly combating demoralization:

1. An emotionally charged, confiding relationship with a helping person, often with the participation of a group
2. A healing setting which heightens the therapist's prestige and strengthens the patient's expectation of help by symbolizing the therapist's role as a healer

3. A rational, conceptual scheme, or myth that provides a plausible explanation for the patient's symptoms and prescribes a ritual or procedure for resolving them

4. A ritual or *procedure* [italics added] that requires active participation of both patient and therapist and that is believed by both to be the means of restoring the patient's health (5, p. 20)

■ APPLICATION OF CULTURAL KNOWLEDGE AND CULTURE-SPECIFIC TECHNIQUES IN THE PROCESSES OF PSYCHOTHERAPY FOR U.S. MINORITY GROUPS

Cross-cultural encounters vividly accentuate the challenge when psychotherapy is applied in different contexts. When one study (14) examined the adequacy of psychotherapeutic services and treatment practices for U.S. ethnic minority groups, minority groups fared quite poorly. In a study (12) of utilization rates by nearly 14,000 clients in 17 community mental health centers in the greater Seattle area, all of the ethnic minority groups had significantly higher dropout rates than Caucasians. It is therefore not surprising that the Special Population Task Force of the President's Commission on Mental Health (15) concluded that ethnic minorities "are clearly underserved or inappropriately served by the current mental health system in this country" (15, p. 73).

Several explanations, including the lack of bilingual therapists, therapists' stereotypes toward ethnic clients, and discrimination were advanced (12). However, as Sue pointed out

the single most important explanation for the problems in service delivery involves the inability of therapists to provide culturally responsive forms of treatment. The assumption, and a fairly good one, is that most therapists are not familiar with the cultural backgrounds and life-styles of various ethnic-minority groups and have received training primarily developed for Anglo, or mainstream, Americans. (12, p. 37)

Clearly, a case can be argued for therapists to increase their cultural sensitiveness and knowledge of their patients. Indeed, in an effort to be more culturally responsive, federal policy makers recommended an increase in the hiring of bilingual and bicultural personnel who could work with ethnic minority patients (12). The issue of therapist-patient fitness in the process of psychotherapy has also been the subject of considerable research (12).

Nonetheless, more recent findings have shown that mere possession of cultural knowledge when applied in inappropriate ways, particularly when this knowledge is quite distal to the goals of psychotherapy, is insufficient (12). The search for appropriate application of cultural knowledge that is linked to particular processes that result in effective psychotherapy led Sue and Zane (12) to examine two basic elements, *credibility* and *giving,* as examples of two important therapeutic variables when working with ethnic clients.

> *Credibility* refers to the client's perception of the therapist as an effective and trustworthy helper. *Giving* is the client's perception that something was received from the therapeutic encounter. . . . *Ascribed status* is the position or role that one is assigned by others. . . . *Achieved credibility* refers more directly to the therapists' skills. (12, p. 40)

Credibility with ethnic patients can be strengthened in at least three ways:

1. Conceptualizing the client's problem in a manner that is congruent with the client's belief systems
2. Providing culturally appropriate means for problem resolution
3. Defining goals that are compatible between therapist and client (12, p. 41)

Symbols and ideas of "gifts" in the therapeutic encounter can include symptom reduction, cognitive clarity, normalization, reassurance, hope and faith, acquisition of skills, increased coping, and appropriate goal setting (12).

In the following case that I have paraphrased, Sue and Morishima cited the example of a culturally sensitive way of encouraging a Chinese client's use of third-party intermediaries to resolve conflicts:

> The case relates to a Chinese housewife immigrant from Hong Kong. Six months after their wedding, her husband invited his parents to move in and stay with them out of a sense of filial obligation. Faced with the demands of her in-laws to serve them and the lack of support she received from her husband, this client became distressed and distraught. During therapy, she was encouraged by her therapist to seek a third-party intermediary to resolve conflict. The enlistment of the older brother of her mother-in-law to intervene came to mind.
>
> On a visit to his sister (client's mother-in-law), her older brother told her that the client "looked unhappy, that possibly she was working too hard, and that she needed a little more praise for the work that she was doing in taking care of everyone." This intervention resulted in a noticeable diminution of the mother-in-law's criticism and it was noted that she had even begun to help the client with household chores. (12)

This case example illustrates how cultural values of respect for elders, face-saving, avoidance of confrontation, and preservation of a harmonious family relationship can be mobilized to resolve conflict through the use of a third-party intermediary.

Similarly, I present the case of a hospitalized elderly depressed Chinese woman I treated, in which I actively mobilized family members as intermediaries in the treatment:

> During a psychiatric consultation regarding an elderly Chinese woman with severe depression at a local hospital in Boston, I noticed the patient refused to talk, drink, or eat. No amount of encouragement from the medical or nursing staff could prevent her from sliding into a very self-destructive, deteriorating course. Electroconvulsive therapy was strongly considered because of the immediate threat to her physical health.

On interview with relatives, I discovered that she had recently had a heart attack shortly after she felt rejected by her son and daughter-in-law when she visited them in New York City. She felt ignored and rejected when she was left alone in her son's apartment because both her son and daughter-in-law had to work during the day. Shortly after she returned to Massachusetts, she developed a myocardial infarction and was literally "heart broken." Her sullenness and refusal to eat betrayed a deep sense of sadness and disappointment.

When I elicited the circumstances of her depression, I contacted her son and conveyed to him the dynamics of her illness and rejection. He immediately brought his whole family to Boston to visit his mother. Profusely apologetic, her son strongly encouraged the patient to drink and eat. After persistent coaxing, the patient finally took the first sip of tea. This small gesture led her to consume meals. Eventually, she was able to pull herself out of a severe depression. Electroconvulsive therapy was averted.

Again, both of these cases illustrate how a patient's cultural values can be effectively used in the process of therapeutic intervention. Further, it illustrates the social context in which healing takes place. In both cases, the restoration of a harmonious family relationship was as an important part of healing as the lifting of the patients' depression.

So far, my discussion of the cultural context of psychotherapy has centered on the *processes* of the psychotherapeutic relationship. I now turn to the examination of the influence of cultural variables on the *structure* of the psychotherapeutic relationship.

■ STRUCTURE OF THE PSYCHOTHERAPEUTIC RELATIONSHIP

Because there are many parallels between the doctor-patient relationship and other forms of the therapist-patient relationship, I use the physician-patient relationship as a paradigm to examine the structure of the whole spectrum of therapeutic relationships. In an international conference held to examine the changing context of the doctor-patient relationship, Bloom and Summey (16) provided a useful model that explicates the basic elements of the nature of the doctor-patient relationship based on a transactional analysis model (Figure 8–1).

The five components of the clinician-patient encounter are 1) the context, 2) the therapist or counselor, 3) the patient or client, 4) the human interaction between the two-person set, and 5) the application of technical information (16). All five of these components are intimately related to the social and cultural background of both the therapist and the patient—their value orientation, mode of interaction, concepts, constructs, and customary procedures that are all components of culture (see Chapter 1, Culture in Psychiatry).

In this model, the following are the key elements:

1. *The doctor and patient interact as a two-person set.* The human interaction and rapport between the two persons rests heavily on the personality attributes of the two individuals and is conveyed as *expressive* transactions. The special knowledge, skills, and procedures imparted in the process of healing between the two persons compose the *instrumental* transaction (16).

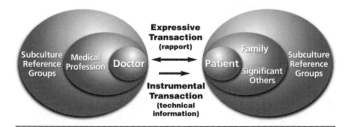

Macrosociocultural Context

Expressive Transaction (rapport)

Instrumental Transaction (technical information)

Subculture Reference Groups — Medical Profession — Doctor ↔ Patient — Family — Significant Others — Subculture Reference Groups

FIGURE 8–1. **Macrocultural context of the doctor-patient relationship.**
Source. Adapted from Bloom SW: *The Doctor and His Patient.* New York, Russell Sage Foundation, 1963, p. 256.

2. *Each individual is also an epitome of his or her culture.* This implies that values, beliefs, concepts, and procedures derived from major subcultural reference groups heavily influence the behavior of the two actors. For the physician, standards for behavior prescribed by the medical profession, including ethical and procedural guidelines that are internalized by the physician, serve as guidelines for medical decision making. For the patient, standards for behavior from dominant subcultural groups, such as the family or a religious sect, frequently dictate medical decisions made by the patient.

3. *Standards for behavior in the larger sociocultural matrix also directly or indirectly influence the transaction between the doctor and patient.* The introduction of a third-party payer system and practice guidelines from federal and state regulatory agencies that prescribe standards for medical practice are prime examples.

Macrosocial Context of the Physician-Patient Relationship

Therapy does not occur in a vacuum. Therapeutic techniques are guided not only by the school of theory therapists subscribe to but also by other contextual factors, often unarticulated, that powerfully operate to influence the therapeutic encounter. As already mentioned, standards for professional reference groups guide physician behavior. As for the patients, the family and significant others often influence the conduct of the individual.

Broad, societal standards for behaviors, often reflecting dominant sociocultural values, promulgated by governmental agencies, though distal to the immediate setting of care, can profoundly influence the behavior of both the professional and the health care institutions.

Consider, for example, standards set by regulatory agencies such as the Joint Commission on Accreditation of Healthcare Organizations and the Health Care Financing Administration. These agencies prescribe values (what constitutes "quality" care), belief (patient's right), procedures, and guidelines for clinical protocol (seclusion and restraint) that must be fulfilled in order for health care institutions to be certified as providing an acceptable level of care.

Models of the Macrosocial Context of the Doctor-Patient Relationship

The onset of the era of managed care in the United States provides a window of opportunity to clarify the impact of the macrosocial context on the physician-patient relationship. In other words, how do the political and economic forces in the macrosocial environment affect the therapist-patient relationship? The impact of this change can be examined through the vicissitudes of changes in the model of the doctor-patient relationship from both a historical and a sociological perspective. As noted, each model reflects important changes in the structure of this relationship.

Earlier Models of the Therapeutic Relationship

Bloom and Summey (16) cited two predominant earlier models of the doctor-patient relationship: a *functionalist-integrated model* and a *structural determinist model.*

Functionalist-integrated model. This model is exemplified by the view of the doctor-patient relationship as a social system. Lawrence J. Henderson, the outstanding American physician well known for his formulation in 1908 of the acid-base equilibrium in the physiological study of blood, and Vilfredo Pareto, a practicing engineer, were credited for first applying system theory to the study of the doctor-patient relationship (16). Subsequently, Talcott Parsons carried forth Henderson's discussion of the doctor-patient relationship and developed it as part of a sociological theory. Parsons regarded the doctor-patient relationship as a social system. Its key premises were the following:

- The problem of health is intimately involved in the functional prerequisites of the social system. Too low a general level of health, too high an incidence of illness, is dysfunctional.

- Sickness and health are, because of their importance, part of the culture.
- Health care is a social role relationship between a helping agent and a person needing help.
- The social roles of the health care relationship are a patterned sector of culture and are thus learned sequences of behavior. (16, pp. 21–22)

The Parsonian model viewed the therapeutic relationship as a functionally integrated system based on a social system concept. (*System* refers to "the concept that refers to both the complex of interdependencies between parts, components, and processes that involves discernible regularities of relationship, and to a similar type of interdependency between such a complex and the surrounding environment" [16, p. 18].)

In this model, the functional prerequisite of the doctor-patient relationship is emphasized. The sick role, albeit involuntary in cause, is conceptualized as a type of social deviance. Patients are thought to socialize into a sick role, whose privileges include exemption from performance of normal social obligations and from responsibility for one's own state. The professional, on the other hand, possessing technical expertise, legitimizes the claim of patients to illness, and is responsible for returning the sick person to his or her normal role in society. In the ideal professional role, the professional is expected to "act for the welfare of the patient, be guided by professional rules for conduct, apply a high degree of achieved skill and knowledge to solve problem of illness, and to maintain objective neutrality in the execution of his/her responsibilities" (16, p. 24). The professional, through the exercise of healing technique, returns the sick person to his or her normal role in society, thus preventing abuses by persons (though no fault of their own) who gain psychological rewards as a result of the legitimized role of dependency of illness. In so doing, professionals also benefit society by exercising a social control responsibility (16). This whole interrelationship connotes the idea of a societal homeostasis from the system point of view.

In the above functionalist model, although the influence of outside socioeconomic forces and culture were recognized, the individual patient was assumed to be the decision maker. The motivations of both the professional and the patient were considered, and individual choice was emphasized. Thus, the functionally integrated system emphasized the social psychological aspect of the professional-patient relationship and was seen as an ideal type of the therapeutic relationship.

Structural determinist model.   More recently, the works of several authors, notably that of Mechanic, Freidson, and others (16), challenged the Parsonian view. These authors emphasized other players in the "role-set," such as the patient's family, nurses, and significant others in the care process (16). Freidson viewed the relationship between the physician and the patient as a "clash of perspective," each seeking to gain his or her own interests from the other or, as Bloom and Summey phrased it, "an encounter between two distinct social systems, and not a functionally contained, homeostatic system in itself" (16, p. 31). Freidson emphasized the "necessity of conflict in human relationships." To Freidson, the fundamental fact is that the physician defines illness and confers the status of patient, "quite apart from the incumbent's motivation" (16, p. 75). The physician determines what is normal and who is sick, an official role conferred by society. The patient is "someone to whom something happens, who is then labeled by others and pressed to behave in a particular expected way quite independently of his own motives or desires. . . . His motives may determine how he performs in that role, but not whether or not he is placed in that role" (16, p. 81). In this sense, Freidson's thinking is akin to the "labeling theory" of Szasz, Scheff, and Goffman (16).

Waitzkin and Waterman (1974) and Navarro (1975) extended the structural analytic and conflict theory into the sociopolitical structure of the society and viewed the doctor-patient relationship as a "typical collectivity" within the institution of medicine (16). "In all societies, health care is a service provided by one group of people (health workers) to another (patients). Society differs greatly, nevertheless, in the ways they organize this service" (16, p. 34). In a capitalist system of care that is organized around profit, as in for-profit health maintenance organizations in the United States, there exists a tension between the need to maintain profit and good health. One group seeks to exploit the other (16).

Current Conception of the Macrosocial Context of the Doctor-Patient Relationship

Currently, Parsons offers four models in the conceptualization of the macrosocial context of the doctor-patient relationship (see Table 8–1). Each model has an admixture of features of the other (17).

The market model. This model regards the patient as a "consumer" with the implications that the health care agent, notably the physician, should be regarded as the "provider," the seller of a service, and that the basis of the relationship is primarily economic. Because health care is a service, it must be financed in some way. Traditionally, the patient paid the servicing agent directly. The injection of third-party organizational payers into the doctor-patient relationship, which have financial interests with the patients, significantly alters the domain of this relationship. Confidentiality and the freedom to exercise the scientific-technical component that requires special knowledge and competence in dealing with the requisite problem, the most important and distinctive feature of this relationship, is altered significantly (17). In this context, the doctor-patient relationship is conceived of as a *pattern* that can be subjected to a "negotiation" (18). However, with the rising educational level of patients and the sentiment of "consumerism," a desire for an increasingly "democratic set of attitudes" sets into motion a demand for a more open inquiry of the bases of medical decisions made by physicians and allied health personnel. There is now a greater challenge to the "authoritarian treatment" of the patients by the "traditional physicians." The patient, as a consumer, now demands adequate explanations of what is done in the name of consumerism.

TABLE 8-1. Models of social organization for health services

Model	Central concerns	Distinguishing features
Market	Health care is a service and must be financed in some way. Basis of the relationship is primarily economic. "Wants" of patients are emphasized.	Patient is regarded as a customer, a "consumer" of a service, and the physician as "provider," the seller of a service.
Bureaucratic organization	Institutionalization of organizational responsibility. Authority is centrally prominent. Included is the notion of "proletarianization" of the medical profession.	Emphasis is on the engineering-technological aspects of care. Employing organization controls the training and education of its key employees. The physician, as salaried employee, increasingly carries out the missions and functions of the employing organization.
Democratic association	"Rights" and equality of the patient in a common membership with the physician are emphasized.	Both patients and physicians are regarded as belonging in the same category as members of an organization who in all fundamental respects should be treated as equals.
Collegial association	Conception of health, illness, and health care is grounded in a complex framework that comprehends the dynamics of both somatic and personality balances and their interdependence.	Professional competence and responsibility are legitimized as prior conditions of entry into the relationship. Though stratified on axes of competence and responsibility, it regards those who share a common status as presumptive equals.

Source. Adapted from reference 17.

The bureaucratic organization model.   This model has predominantly administrative functions akin to that of tax collection. Closely related is the notion of the *proletarianization* of the medical profession, a process by which the medical profession is gradually "divested of control over certain prerogatives relating to location, content, and essentiality of its task activities and is hereby subordinated to the broader requirements of production under advanced capitalism." (19, p. 158). The replacement of the mode of financing health care within the traditional fee-for-service private practice by large-scale financing organizations introduced the element of a bureaucracy. Many physicians are now salaried employees of organizations and must ensure the bottom-line economic survival of their employing institutions. The employing organization's prerogatives, mission, and fee-collecting procedures may assume a greater importance and consume more of the physician's time than the practice of medicine. At times, organizational prerogatives may be at variance with the traditional values of the practice of medicine. For example, in both private and public psychiatric institutions, physicians are increasingly being called upon to treat mentally ill criminal offenders and to ensure "safety" of patients in the community, a traditional role of police and legal agencies. Thus, rather than just acting as "guardians of health," the psychiatric physician's role is increasingly enlarged to assume the societal role of "guardians of safety." For example, in planning for discharges of psychiatric patients into the community, patient discharge plans have increasingly had to address issues of ensuing patient and societal safety, in addition to traditional amelioration of psychiatric symptoms.

The democratic association model.   This model focuses on the responsibility of governments to their constituencies and on the organization of voluntary organizations. Based on the premise of "one member, one vote," the assumption is that physicians and patients should be regarded as belonging to the same category as members of an organization and should be treated as such. Patients' rights are emphasized. Physicians' services and medical treatments require *voluntary* consent by patients.

The collegial association model. Though not explicitly stated, Parsons sees this model as embodying certain elements that must be recognized in any conceptualization of the doctor-patient relationship. Implied in Parsons's discussion are the notions of the professional role of physicians, the microsocial aspect and intimacy of the patient-doctor relationship, and the superior role ascribed through technical and knowledge competence of the physician. It is clearly differentiated from the ordinary expectation of patients in their role as buyers of commercial products. It deals with the immediacy of the "existential" problems that attend to an individual's life, its anxieties, death, and other human tragedies (17).

Clinicians and psychotherapists in the current health care environment most likely can identify with some or many of the nuances mentioned above. In fact, such threats to economic survival and freedom of practice of professionals increasingly are putting pressure on professionals to band together to negotiate effectively with third-party payers.

■ BRIDGING THE SOCIOSOMATIC GAP

Germane to the issue of psychotherapy is how words and relationships heal. How can sociocultural variables be integrated with physiological processes? How does the mechanism of psychological healing play out at both the interpersonal level and the microphysiological level? In a series of recent papers, psychiatrist-anthropologist Arthur Kleinman and his colleagues at the Department of Social Medicine at Harvard Medical School have advanced a paradigm of "sociosomatic medicine" in an attempt to bridge the conceptual gap between the macrosocial and microbiological processes (20). They define this method as follows:

A sociosomatic approach encompasses not only the integration of social context into psychosomatic approaches—that is, enhancing the understanding of mind-body interaction to mind-body interactions in context—but it also posits a direct impact of social processes on the body that is outside of the mediation of conscious awareness. (20, p. 291)

Implicit in this model is the suggestion that healing relationships affect psychophysiological processes. However, pathways for healing need to be elucidated that translate changes from the interpersonal to the microphysiological level.

Although we still await unequivocal biological data to conclusively demonstrate the power of this relationship and its therapeutic value, the availability of modern technological investigative tools makes the possibility of this area of investigation distinctly promising.

I believe Kleinman provided a useful paradigm for looking at the therapeutic aspect of this relationship. He proposed a series of stages in the healing process to connect aspects of symbolic healing and cultural meanings with *psychophysiological* structural changes. The four stages Kleinman proposed are as follows:

Stage I: Symbolic linkage between personal experience, social relations, and cultural meanings. Kleinman posited that the first stage of symbolic healing is the presence of sociosomatic linkage between broad cultural symbol systems and meanings in social relations, with psychophysiological codes for communicating at cellular, psychological, and behavioral levels (7). Healing rituals, whether through elicitation of catharsis, trance, or induced feeling of hope and faith, reverse pathophysiological processes that cause the symptomatologies of disturbed functions.

The experiences of individuals in society (e.g., serious loss or misfortune) are signs whose meanings link up with a group's master symbols (e.g., *yin/yang*, the crucified Christ, or the body/self as a broken machine). Those symbols are the deep cultural grammar governing how the person orients himself to the world around him and to his inner world. That cultural grammar is found in the central myths (e.g., the Koran or the Constitution) that authorize the values of the group and that serves as a template for the personal myths of the individual. There is a hierarchy of linked systems running from cultural symbols to social relations and on to self and bodily processes. That hierarchy is the biopsychocultural basis for healing: it underwrites the "upward" assimilation of personal experience into cultural meanings and the "downward" particularization of those meanings into bodily processes via the cognition and affect of a particular person in a particular situation. (7, p. 132)

Stage II: The symbolic connection is activated for a particular person through contact with a healer. Problems from which the patient is suffering are redefined in terms of the authorizing system of cultural meaning (e.g., depressive affects are results of neurochemical changes and therefore can be treated with antidepressants). The patient accepts the redefinition of the problem offered by the healer, thereby aligning his or her distressing experiences with the symbolic values of the healing system. A switching of the communicative codes ensues (from early morning awakening to depression or auditory hallucinations to thought disorder).

Stage III: The skillful guidance of therapeutic change in the patient's emotional reaction through mediating symbols is particularized from the general meaning system. In an atmosphere of mutual expectations conveyed through the clinical reality of the therapeutic interaction, the therapist's interpretations are taken as symbols that are authorized, negotiated, and deeply felt.

Stage IV: The healer confirms the transformation of the particularized symbolic meanings through specific rituals (e.g., exorcism for spirit possession, analysis of transference reactions in therapy). This symbolic transformation juxtaposes cultural symbolic codes and social relations and psychobiology and fosters a desired change in the patient's emotions, disordered physiology, and social ties that eventually leads to an affirmation of success. Kleinman regards this transformation as a work of culture, "the making over of psychophysiological process into meaningful experience and the affirmation of success" (7, p. 134).

What Kleinman proposes is a structural schema to connect symbolic healing with psychophysiological phenomena. In a way, the above schema shares several common therapeutic features of the psychotherapy articulated by Frank and Sue, mentioned earlier in this chapter. It also reflects a restoration of a level of integration of what Engel would ascribe as *cultural* in the overall biopsychosocial schema of an individual homeostatic mechanism (21). Healing imparts a sense of restoration of meaningfulness, a renewed sense of connectedness with the culturally authorized value systems. The individual senses a "wholesome" feeling again because the meaning that binds and drives a person's activities is restored. A transformation of experience has taken place.

■ TOWARD A COMPARATIVE PARADIGM FOR THE ANALYSIS OF THE CULTURAL CONTEXT OF PSYCHOTHERAPY

Given the various macrosocial and cultural contexts that affect the therapeutic relationship, is there a way to conceptualize therapeutic encounters cross-culturally? Kleinman aptly pointed out that psychotherapists who study healing are so preoccupied with the content of particular kinds of healing systems and with proving that a particular mechanism of change is universal that they miss out on the key contribution of culture: *symbolic healing*. He asserted that "it is the structural organization of healing on the level of *symbolic meanings* that unified all healing systems, psychotherapy included" (7, p. 136).

In an attempt to provide a comparative paradigm for the understanding and study of psychotherapy in various cultural systems, Kleinman proposes a model of analysis that has heuristic application for clinical care, teaching, and research. As an example of its application, depending on the dominant cultural value, psychotherapy can be posited to occur according to two basic approaches: a more individual, person-centered approach or a more sociocentric approach. Table 8–2 compares the context of these two approaches.

The above paradigm provides a conceptual framework that can be used to teach, learn, and research psychotherapy in a cross-cultural context. By first exploring the structural model of healing, one can then review what is known about universal and culture-specific aspects of symbolic healing, including psychotherapy (7).

TABLE 8–2. **Comparison of egocentric (psychodynamically oriented) psychotherapy and sociocentric (folk) psychotherapy**

Criteria	Egocentric (psychodynamic)	Sociocentric (folk)
1. Institutional setting	Professional institution	Folk arena
2. Characteristics of the interpersonal interaction		
• Number of participants	Usually dyadic	Multiple, including family
• Time coordinate	Continuous	Episodic
• Quality of the relationship	Formal, egalitarian, private	Informal, authoritarian, public
3. Characteristics of the practitioners		
• Personality	Warm, empathic	Charismatic
• Training	Formal	Informal
• Type of practice	Special interests and skills	General
• Rewards	Monetary	Monetary and/or materials
4. Idioms of communication		
• Mode	Psychological	Religious/moral
• Treatment negotiation	Open, egalitarian	Tacit, authoritarian
5. Clinical reality		
• Sacred or secular	Secular	Sacred
• Disease/illness orientation	Disease/illness	Illness
• Focus of treatment	Individual	Familial, group
• Patient- or practitioner-centered	Patient	Practitioner

	Mix	Symbolic
• Symbolic and/or instrumental intervention		
• Therapeutic expectations	Long term, modest	Immediate, substantial
• Insight as an ingredient of therapeutic change	Expected	Not expected
• Treatment goals	Individuation, personal growth	Group harmony, integration with family
• Perceived locus of responsibility for care	Patient	Family
• Confession and moral witnessing	Expected and witnessed	May be expected and witnessed
6. Therapeutic stages and mechanisms		
• Process	Fostering of therapeutic alliance, analysis of transference and countertransference issues, endorsement of personality change	Symbolic therapy such as exorcism; personality change not endorsed
• Mechanisms	Catharsis, social learning and conditioning, persuasion, behavioral control, altered state of consciousness (hypnosis, relaxation) of patient, sense of mastery, insight	Catharsis, persuasion, remoralization, altered state of consciousness (trance and possession) of shaman, practical problem solving, clarification, explanation, sense of mastery

(continued)

TABLE 8–2. **Comparison of egocentric (psychodynamically oriented) psychotherapy and sociocentric (folk) psychotherapy** *(continued)*

• Adherence to prescribed treatments and prescribed activities	Present	Present
• Termination	Significant issue	Insignificant issue
• Evaluation of outcome	Considerable studies	Few studies
7. Extratherapeutic aspects		
• Social control	Control exerted through the application of technical interventions and social authority	Control exerted through community consensus
• Ethical codes	Formal codes holding healers accountable	No formal code to hold healers accountable
• Economic costs and constraints on access	Found cost-effective in reducing overutilization of primary care services and hospitalization, treatment of common psychiatric problems (depression, anxiety) and "life problems" (marital, midlife crises, adolescent turmoil). Governmental financing of psychosocial services available; access of poor to professionals problematic	Cost-effectiveness uncertain and unstudied. No governmental financing of psychosocial service. Access of poor to healers may also be problematic.
• Political implications	May challenge orthodox definitions of reality	May challenge orthodox definitions of reality

Source. Adapted from reference 7.

■ IMPLICATIONS FOR PSYCHOTHERAPISTS AND COUNSELORS

1. *Psychotherapy is culture-bound.* Both the patients and the therapists are the epitome of their unique cultural heritage. It behooves therapists to consciously explicate their own cultural concepts, constructs, beliefs, values, and operational procedures and examine how these can be brought to bear upon the therapeutic encounter.

2. *Transference and countertransference issues may be accentuated in the cross-cultural encounter.* Cross-cultural counseling is a demanding and involving experience and may intensify the therapist's countertransference experiences. Likewise, the transference feelings of helplessness, ambiguity, and dependence frequently experienced by patients seeking psychotherapy may also be exacerbated in a new cultural milieu. Thus, the contribution of culture in the intensification of the personal experience adds to the demands placed on the counselor when therapy is conducted across the gulf of culture (11).

3. *Therapists must be cognizant and attentive to micro- as well as macrosocial issues that influence both the process and the structural elements of the clinician-patient relationship.* Unless one is practicing on a strictly fee-for-service basis, the introduction of a third-party payer into the context of the therapeutic relationship means that practitioners of psychotherapy must be prepared to meet the challenges of potential intrusion of bureaucratic demands.

4. *There is a great need to systematically examine and research issues pertaining to cross-cultural psychotherapy.* Cross-cultural psychotherapy accentuates what anthropologists long ago discovered: the power of *symbolic healing* in all levels of the healing system. We need to understand both the processes of therapy and the systems within which those processes occur (7).

■ CONCLUSION

The process and structure of psychotherapy, particularly the central aspect of the clinician-patient relationship, are examined within a cultural context. Elements in the broad macrosocial and cultural context that affect the psychotherapeutic relationship are highlighted. Psychotherapists practicing in an increasingly diverse society not only should be cognizant of cultural variables affecting their interaction with their patients, but also should learn the application of key cultural factors that can maximize the therapeutic process. Recent anthropological advances in conceptual understanding of symbolic healing, a feature of culture, can provide a useful framework to begin integrating macrosocial variables and microphysiological processes in the process of healing induced by psychotherapy. It is hoped that through research in cross-cultural psychotherapy, a universal paradigm for an integrated biopsychocultural healing can be achieved.

■ REFERENCES

1. Wohl J: Intercultural psychotherapy: issues, questions, and reflections, in Counseling Across Cultures. Edited by Pederson PB, Draguns JG, Lonner WJ, et al. Honolulu, HI, University Press of Hawaii, 1981, pp 135–138
2. Pederson PB, Draguns JG, Lonner WJ, et al (eds): Counseling Across Cultures. Honolulu, HI, University Press of Hawaii, 1981
3. Opler ME: Some points of comparison and contrast between the treatment of functional disorders by Apache Shamans and modern psychiatric practice. Am J Psychiatry 92:1371–1387, 1936
4. Murphy JM: Psychotherapeutic aspects of Shamanism on St. Lawrence Island, Alaska, in Magic, Faith, and Healing. Edited by Kiev A. New York, Free Press, 1964, pp 53–83
5. Frank JD: Therapeutic components shared by all psychotherapies, in Psychotherapy Research and Behavior Change (Mas-

ter Lecture Series, Vol 1). Edited by Harvey JH, Parks MM. Washington, DC, American Psychological Association, 1982, pp 9–37

6. Frank JD: Psychotherapy, rhetoric, and hermeneutics: implications for practice and research. Psychotherapy 24:293–302, 1987

7. Kleinman A: Rethinking Psychiatry. New York, Free Press, 1988

8. Kluckhohn C, Murray HA: Personality formation: the determinants, in Personality in Nature, Society and Culture. Edited by Kluckhohn C, Murray HA, Schneider DM. New York, Random House/Alfred A. Knopf, 1953, pp 53–65

9. La Barre W: Confession as cathartic therapy in American tribes, in Magic, Faith, and Healing. Edited by Kiev A. New York, Free Press, 1964, pp 36–49

10. Sundberg ND: Research and research hypotheses about effectiveness in intercultural counseling, in Counseling Across Cultures. Edited by Pedersen PP, Draguns JG, Lonner WJ, et al. Honolulu, HI, University Press of Hawaii, 1981, pp 304–342

11. Draguns JG: Counseling across cultures: common themes and distinct approaches, in Counseling Across Cultures. Edited by Pedersen PP, Draguns JG, Lonner WJ, et al. Honolulu, HI, University Press of Hawaii, 1981, pp 1–21

12. Sue S, Zane N: The role of culture and cultural techniques in psychotherapy. Am Psychol 42:37–45, 1987

13. Fisher AR, Jome LM: Reconceptualing multicultural counseling: universal healing conditions in a culturally specific context. Counseling Psychologist 26:525–588, 1998

14. Sue S: Community mental health services to minority groups: some optimism, some pessimism. Am Psychol 32:616–624, 1977

15. Special Populations Task Force of the President's Commission on Mental Health: Task Panel Reports Submitted to the President's Commission on Mental Health, Vol 3. Washington, DC, U.S. Government Printing Office, 1978

16. Bloom SW, Summey S: Models of the doctor-patient relationship: a history of the social system concept, in The Doctor-Patient Relationship in the Changing Health Scene (DHEW Publ No NIH-78–183). Proceedings of the International Conference, April 26–28, 1976, Washington, DC, U.S. Department of Health, Education, and Welfare, Public Health Service, National Institutes of Health, 1976, pp 17–41

17. Parsons T: Epilogue, in The Doctor-Patient Relationship in the Changing Health Scene (DHEW Publ No NIH-78–183). Proceedings of the International Conference, April 26–28, 1976, Washington, DC, U.S. Department of Health, Education, and Welfare, Public Health Service, National Institutes of Health, 1976, pp 445–455

18. Lazare A, Eisenthal S, Wasserman L: The customer approach to patienthood: attending to patient requests in a walk-in clinic. Arch Gen Psychiatry 32:553–558, 1975

19. McKinlay JB: The changing political and economic context of the patient-physician encounter, in The Doctor-Patient Relationship in the Changing Health Scene (DHEW Publ No NIH-78–183), Proceedings of the International Conference, April 26–28, 1976. Washington, DC, U.S. Department of Health, Education, and Welfare, Public Health Service, National Institutes of Health, 1976, pp 155–188

20. Kleinman A, Becker AE: "Sociosomatic": the contributions of anthropology to psychosomatic medicine. Psychosom Med 60:389–457, 1998

21. Engel GL: The clinical application of the biopsychosocial model. Am J Psychotherapy 137:535–544, 1980

Appendix A

GLOSSARY OF CULTURE-BOUND SYNDROMES IN DSM-IV

The term *culture-bound syndrome* denotes recurrent, locality-specific patterns of aberrant behavior and troubling experience that may or may not be linked to a particular DSM-IV diagnostic category. Many of these patterns are indigenously considered to be "illnesses," or at least afflictions, and most have local names. Although presentations conforming to the major DSM-IV categories can be found throughout the world, the particular symptoms, course, and social response are very often influenced by local cultural factors. In contrast, culture-bound syndromes are generally limited to specific societies or culture areas and are localized, folk diagnostic categories that frame coherent meanings for certain repetitive, patterned, and troubling sets of experiences and observations.

There is seldom a one-to-one equivalence of any culture-bound syndrome with a DSM diagnostic entity. Aberrant behavior that might be sorted by a diagnostician using DSM-IV into several categories may be included in a single folk category, and presentations that might be considered by a diagnostician using DSM-IV as belonging to a single category may be sorted into several by an indigenous clinician. Moreover, some conditions and disorders have

Reprinted from American Psychiatric Association: *Diagnostic and Statistical Manual of Mental Disorders*, 4th Edition, Text Revision. Washington, DC, American Psychiatric Association, 2000, pp. 898–903. Used with permission. Copyright 2000, American Psychiatric Association.

been conceptualized as culture-bound syndromes specific to industrialized culture (e.g., anorexia nervosa, dissociative identity disorder) given their apparent rarity or absence in other cultures. It should also be noted that all industrialized societies include distinctive subcultures and widely diverse immigrant groups who may present with culture-bound syndromes.

This glossary lists some of the best-studied culture-bound syndromes and idioms of distress that may be encountered in clinical practice in North America and includes relevant DSM-IV categories when data suggest that they should be considered in a diagnostic formulation.

Amok   A dissociative episode characterized by a period of brooding followed by an outburst of violent, aggressive, or homicidal behavior directed at people and objects. The episode tends to be precipitated by a perceived slight or insult and seems to be prevalent only among males. The episode is often accompanied by persecutory ideas, automatism, amnesia, exhaustion, and a return to the premorbid state following the episode. Some instances of amok may occur during a brief psychotic episode or constitute the onset or an exacerbation of a chronic psychotic process. The original reports that used this term were from Malaysia. A similar behavior pattern is found in Laos, Philippines, Polynesia (*cafard* or *cathard*), Papua New Guinea, and Puerto Rico (*mal de pelea*), and among the Navajo (*iich'aa*).

Ataque de nervios   An idiom of distress principally reported among Latinos from the Caribbean but recognized among many Latin American and Latin Mediterranean groups. Commonly reported symptoms include uncontrollable shouting, attacks of crying, trembling, heat in the chest rising into the head, and verbal or physical aggression. Dissociative experiences, seizurelike or fainting episodes, and suicidal gestures are prominent in some attacks but absent in others. A general feature of an *ataque de nervios* is a sense of being out of control. *Ataques de nervios* frequently occur as a direct result of a stressful event relating to the family (e.g., news of the death of a close relative, a separation or divorce from a spouse, conflicts with a spouse or children, or witnessing an accident involving a family member). People may experience amnesia for what occurred during the *ataque de nervios,* but they otherwise return rapidly to their usual level of functioning. Although descriptions of some *ataques de nervios* most closely fit with the DSM-IV description of panic attacks, the association of most *ataques* with a precipitating event and the frequent absence of the hallmark symptoms of acute fear or apprehension distinguish them from panic disorder. *Ataques* span the range from normal expressions of distress not associated with having a mental disorder to symptom presentations associated with the diagnoses of anxiety, mood, dissociative, or somatoform disorders.

Bilis and **colera** (also referred to as *muina*) The underlying cause of these syndromes is thought to be strongly experienced anger or rage. Anger is viewed among many Latino groups as a particularly powerful emotion that can have direct effects on the body and can exacerbate existing symptoms. The major effect of anger is to disturb core body balances (which are understood as a balance between hot and cold valences in the body and between the material and spiritual aspects of the body). Symptoms can include acute nervous tension, headache, trembling, screaming, stomach disturbances, and in more severe cases, loss of consciousness. Chronic fatigue may result from the acute episode.

Boufée delirante A syndrome observed in West Africa and Haiti. This French term refers to a sudden outburst of agitated and aggressive behavior, marked confusion, and psychomotor excitement. It may sometimes be accompanied by visual and auditory hallucinations or paranoid ideation. These episodes may resemble an episode of brief psychotic disorder.

Brain fag A term initially used in West Africa to refer to a condition experienced by high school or university students in response to the challenges of schooling. Symptoms include difficulties in concentrating, remembering, and thinking. Students often state that their brains are "fatigued." Additional somatic symptoms are usually centered around the head and neck and include pain, pressure or tightness, blurring of vision, heat, or burning. "Brain tiredness" or fatigue from "too much thinking" is an idiom of distress in many cultures, and resulting syndromes can resemble certain anxiety, depressive, and somatoform disorders.

Dhat A folk diagnostic term used in India to refer to severe anxiety and hypochondriacal concerns associated with the discharge of semen, whitish discoloration of the urine, and feelings of weakness and exhaustion. Similar to *jiryan* (India), *sukra prameha* (Sri Lanka), and *shen-k'uei* (China).

Falling-out or **blacking out** These episodes occur primarily in southern United States and Caribbean groups. They are characterized by a sudden collapse, which sometimes occurs without warning but sometimes is preceded by feelings of dizziness or "swimming" in the head. The individual's eyes are usually open, but the person claims an inability to see. The person usually hears and understands what is occurring around him or her but feels powerless to move. This may correspond to a diagnosis of conversion disorder or a dissociative disorder.

Ghost sickness A preoccupation with death and the deceased (sometimes associated with witchcraft) frequently observed among members of many American Indian tribes. Various symptoms can be attributed to ghost sickness, including bad dreams, weakness, feelings of danger, loss of appetite, fainting, dizziness, fear, anxiety, hallucinations, loss of consciousness, confusion, feelings of futility, and a sense of suffocation.

hwa-byung (also known as *wool-hwa-byung*) A Korean folk syndrome literally translated into English as "anger syndrome" and attributed to the suppression of anger. The symptoms include insomnia, fatigue, panic, fear of impending death, dysphoric affect, indigestion, anorexia, dyspnea, palpitations, generalized aches and pains, and a feeling of a mass in the epigastrium.

koro A term, probably of Malaysian origin, that refers to an episode of sudden and intense anxiety that the penis (or, in females, the vulva and nipples) will recede into the body and possibly cause death. The syndrome is reported in south and east Asia, where it is known by a variety of local terms such as *shuk yang, shook yong,* and *suo yang* (Chinese); *jinjinia bemar* (Assam); or *rok-joo* (Thailand). It is occasionally found in the West. Koro at times occurs in localized epidemic form in east Asian areas. This diagnosis is included in the *Chinese Classification of Mental Disorders,* Second Edition (CCMD-2).

Latah   Hypersensitivity to sudden fright, often with echopraxia, echolalia, command obedience, and dissociative or trancelike behavior. The term *latah* is of Malaysian or Indonesian origin, but the syndrome has been found in many parts of the world. Other terms for this condition are *amurakh, irkunii, ikota, olan, myriachit,* and *menkeiti* (Siberian groups); *bah tschi, bah-tsi, baah-ji* (Thailand); *imu* (Ainu, Sakhalin, Japan); and *mali-mali* and *silok* (Philippines). In Malaysia it is more frequent in middle-aged women.

Locura   A term used by Latinos in the United States and Latin America to refer to a severe form of chronic psychosis. The condition is attributed to an inherited vulnerability, to the effect of multiple life difficulties, or to a combination of both factors. Symptoms exhibited by persons with *locura* include incoherence, agitation, auditory and visual hallucinations, inability to follow rules of social interaction, unpredictability, and possible violence.

Mal de ojo   A concept widely found in Mediterranean cultures and elsewhere in the world. *Mal de ojo* is a Spanish phrase translated into English as "evil eye." Children are especially at risk. Symptoms include fitful sleep, crying without apparent cause, diarrhea, vomiting, and fever in a child or infant. Sometimes adults (especially females) have the condition.

Nervios   A common idiom of distress among Latinos in the United States and Latin America. A number of other ethnic groups have related, though often somewhat distinctive, ideas of "nerves" (such as *nevra* among Greeks in North America). *Nervios* refers both to a general state of vulnerability to stressful life experiences and to a syndrome brought on by difficult life circumstances. The term *nervios* includes a wide range of symptoms of emotional distress, somatic disturbance, and inability to function. Common symptoms include headaches and "brain aches," irritability, stomach disturbances, sleep difficulties, nervousness, easy tearfulness, inability to concentrate, trembling, tingling sensations, and *mareos* (dizziness with occasional vertigo-like exacerbations). *Nervios* tends to be an ongoing problem, although variable in the degree of disability manifested. *Nervios* is a very broad syndrome that spans the range from cases free of a mental disorder to presentations resembling adjustment, anxiety, depressive, dissociative, somatoform, or psychotic disorders. Differential diagnosis will depend on the constellation of symptoms experienced, the kind of social events that are associated with the onset and progress of *nervios,* and the level of disability experienced.

Pibloktoq   An abrupt dissociative episode accompanied by extreme excitement of up to 30 minutes' duration and frequently followed by convulsive seizures and coma lasting up to 12 hours. This is observed primarily in arctic and subarctic Eskimo communities, although regional variations in name exist. The individual may be withdrawn or mildly irritable for a period of hours or days before the attack and will typically report complete amnesia for the attack. During the attack, the individual may tear off his or her clothing, break furniture, shout obscenities, eat feces, flee from protective shelters, or perform other irrational or dangerous acts.

Qi-gong psychotic reaction   A term describing an acute, time-limited episode characterized by dissociative, paranoid, or other psychotic or nonpsychotic symptoms that may occur after participation in the Chinese folk health-enhancing practice of *qi-gong* ("exercise of vital energy"). Especially vulnerable are individuals who become overly involved in the practice. This diagnosis is included in the *Chinese Classification of Mental Disorders,* Second Edition (CCMD-2).

Rootwork   A set of cultural interpretations that ascribes illness to hexing, witchcraft, sorcery, or the evil influence of another person. Symptoms may include generalized anxiety and gastrointestinal complaints (e.g., nausea, vomiting, diarrhea), weakness, dizziness, the fear of being poisoned, and sometimes fear of being killed ("voodoo death"). "Roots," "spells," or "hexes" can be "put," or placed, on other persons, causing a variety of emotional and psychological problems. The "hexed" person may even fear death until the "root" has been "taken off" (eliminated), usually through the work of a "root doctor" (a healer in this tradition), who can also be called on to bewitch an enemy. *Rootwork* is found in the southern United States among both African American and European American populations and in Caribbean societies. It is also known as *mal puesto* or *brujeria* in Latino societies.

Sangue dormido ("sleeping blood") This syndrome is found among Portuguese Cape Verde Islanders (and immigrants from there to the United States) and includes pain, numbness, tremor, paralysis, convulsions, stroke, blindness, heart attack, infection, and miscarriage.

Shenjing shuairuo ("neurasthenia") In China, a condition characterized by physical and mental fatigue, dizziness, headaches, other pains, concentration difficulties, sleep disturbance, and memory loss. Other symptoms include gastrointestinal problems, sexual dysfunction, irritability, excitability, and various signs suggesting disturbance of the autonomic nervous system. In many cases, the symptoms would meet the criteria for a DSM-IV mood or anxiety disorder. This diagnosis is included in the *Chinese Classification of Mental Disorders,* Second Edition (CCMD-2).

Shen-k'uei (Taiwan), **shenkui** (China) A Chinese folk label describing marked anxiety or panic symptoms with accompanying somatic complaints for which no physical cause can be demonstrated. Symptoms include dizziness, backache, fatigability, general weakness, insomnia, frequent dreams, and complaints of sexual dysfunction (such as premature ejaculation and impotence). Symptoms are attributed to excessive semen loss from frequent intercourse, masturbation, nocturnal emission, or passing of "white turbid urine" believed to contain semen. Excessive semen loss is feared because of the belief that it represents the loss of one's vital essence and can thereby be life threatening.

Shin-byung   A Korean folk label for a syndrome in which initial phases are characterized by anxiety and somatic complaints (general weakness, dizziness, fear, anorexia, insomnia, gastrointestinal problems), with subsequent dissociation and possession by ancestral spirits.

Spell   A trance state in which individuals "communicate" with deceased relatives or with spirits. At times this state is associated with brief periods of personality change. This culture-specific syndrome is seen among African Americans and European Americans from the southern United States. Spells are not considered to be medical events in the folk tradition but may be misconstrued as psychotic episodes in clinical settings.

Susto   ("fright" or "soul loss") A folk illness prevalent among some Latinos in the United States and among people in Mexico, Central America, and South America. *Susto* is also referred to as *espanto, pasmo, tripa ida, perdida del alma,* or *chibih. Susto* is an illness attributed to a frightening event that causes the soul to leave the body and results in unhappiness and sickness. Individuals with *susto* also experience significant strains in key social roles. Symptoms may appear any time from days to years after the fright is experienced. It is believed that in extreme cases, *susto* may result in death. Typical symptoms include appetite disturbances, inadequate or excessive sleep, troubled sleep or dreams, feeling of sadness, lack of motivation to do anything, and feelings of low self-worth or dirtiness. Somatic symptoms accompanying *susto* include muscle aches and pains, headache, stomachache, and diarrhea. Ritual healings are focused on calling the soul back to the body and cleansing the person to restore bodily and spiritual balance. Different experiences of *susto* may be related to major depressive disorder, posttraumatic stress disorder, and somatoform disorders. Similar etiological beliefs and symptom configurations are found in may parts of the world.

Taijin kyofusho   A culturally distinctive phobia in Japan, in some ways resembling social phobia in DSM-IV. This syndrome refers to an individual's intense fear that his or her body, its parts or its functions, displease, embarrass, or are offensive to other people in appearance, odor, facial expressions, or movements. This syndrome is included in the official Japanese diagnostic system for mental disorders.

Zar   A general term applied in Ethiopia, Somalia, Egypt, Sudan, Iran, and other North African and Middle Eastern societies to the experience of spirits possessing an individual. Persons possessed by a spirit may experience dissociative episodes that may include shouting, laughing, hitting the head against a wall, singing, or weeping. Individuals may show apathy and withdrawal, refusing to eat or carry out daily tasks, or may develop a long-term relationship with the possessing spirit. Such behavior is not considered pathological locally.

Appendix B

ANNOTATED BIBLIOGRAPHY ON CULTURAL PSYCHIATRY AND RELATED TOPICS

*Akhtar S: Immigration and Identity, Turmoil, Treatment, and Transformation. Northvale, NJ, Jason Aronson, 1999. *Outstanding overview mainly along diagnostic categories.*

*Alarcon R (ed): Cultural psychiatry. Psychiatr Clin N Am 18:3, 1995. *Outstanding overview mainly along diagnostic categories.*

**Alarcon RD, Foulks EF, Vakkur M: Personality Disorders and Culture: Clinical and Conceptual Interactions. New York, Wiley, 1998. *An immediate classic.*

American Medical Association: Cultural Competence Compendium. Chicago, IL, American Medical Association, 1999

American Psychiatric Association: Ethnic Minority Elderly: A Task Force Report of the American Psychiatric Association. Washington, DC, American Psychiatric Association, 1994

Association of American Medical Colleges: Medical School Objectives Project, Parts I–III. Washington, DC, Association of American Medical Colleges, 1998, 1999

Berzoff J, Flanagan LM, Hertz P: Inside Out and Outside In. Northvale, NJ, Jason Aronson, 1996. *Discusses impact of cultural identity variables (race, gender, class, etc.) on psychotherapy.*

This bibliography is courtesy of Francis G. Lu, M.D.

*Denotes a useful book for teaching.

**Denotes an essential core textbook.

Boehnlein JK (ed): Psychiatry and Religion: The Convergence of Mind and Spirit. Washington, DC, American Psychiatric Association, 2000. *An important update on issues at the interface.*

Boorstein S: Clinical Studies in Transpersonal Psychotherapy. Albany, NY, State University of New York Press, 1997

Bynum B: The African Unconscious. New York, Teachers College Press, 1999

**Cabaj R, Stein T (eds): Textbook of Homosexuality and Mental Health. Washington, DC, American Psychiatric Press, 1996. *Very comprehensive. The standard textbook in this area.*

*Canino I, Spurlock J: Culturally Diverse Children and Adolescents. New York, Guilford, 2000. *Practical guidelines.*

*Carter R: The Influence of Race and Racial Identity in Psychotherapy. New York, Wiley, 1995. *Focuses comprehensively on race and psychotherapy.*

*Castillo R: Culture and Mental Illness: A Client Centered Approach. Pacific Grove, CA, Brooks/Cole, 1997. *Discusses assessment, therapy, and cultural issues within diagnostic categories.*

Castillo RJ (ed): Meanings of Madness. Pacific Grove, CA, Brooks/Cole, 1998

*Center for Mental Health Services Substance Abuse and Mental Health Services Administration: Cultural Competence Standards in Managed Care Mental Health Services for Four Underserved/Underrepresented Racial/Ethnic Groups. Washington, DC, Center for Mental Health Services Substance Abuse and Mental Health Services Administration, 1998. *Essential for understanding systems cultural competence.*

*Center for Substance Abuse Treatment/Substance Abuse and Mental Health Services Administration: Cultural Issues in Substance Abuse Treatment. Washington, DC, CSAT/Substance Abuse and Mental Health Services Administration, 1999. *An outstanding monograph on substance abuse.*

**Comas-Diaz L, Greene B (eds): Women of Color: Integrating Ethnic and Gender Identities in Psychotherapy. New York, Guilford, 1994. *The best textbook on this topic.*

*Comas-Diaz L, Griffith E (eds): Clinical Guidelines in Cross-Cultural Mental Health. New York, Wiley, 1988

Dana RH: Multicultural Assessment Perspectives for Professional Psychology. Boston, MA, Allyn & Bacon, 1993

*Dana RH: Understanding Cultural Identity in Intervention and Assessment. Thousand Oaks, CA, Sage, 1997

Desjarlais R, Eisenberg L, Good B, et al: World Mental Health. New York, Oxford University Press, 1995. *Well-researched exposition on the major challenges in global mental health.*

Ewalt PL, Freeman EM, Kirk SA, et al (eds): Multicultural Issues in Social Work. Washington, DC, NASW Press, 1997

*Fadiman A: The Spirit Catches You and You Fall Down. New York, Noonday Press, 1997. *An extraordinary story about the importance of cultural competence in medical care.*

*Foster RP, Moskowitz M, Javier RA (eds): Reaching Across Boundaries of Culture and Class: Widening the Scope of Psychotherapy. Northvale, NJ, Jason Aronson, 1996

**Friedman S (ed): Cultural Issues in the Treatment of Anxiety. New York, Guilford, 1997. *Essential reading for those treating anxiety disorders.*

Fukuyama MA, Sevig TD: Integrating Spirituality Into Multicultural Counseling. Thousand Oaks, CA, Sage, 1999

Garcia J, Zea M (eds): Psychological Interventions and Research With Latino Populations. Boston, MA, Allyn and Bacon, 1997

Gardiner HW, Mutter JD, Kosmitzki C: Lives Across Culture: Cross Cultural Human Development. Boston, MA, Allyn and Bacon, 1998

***Gaw A (ed): Culture, Ethnicity, and Mental Illness. Washington, DC, American Psychiatric Press, 1993. *Comprehensive overview, organized by ethnic minority group.*

Gibbs JT, Huang L (eds): Children of Color: Psychological Interventions With Culturally Diverse Youth, Revised. San Francisco, CA, Jossey-Bass, 1997

Goldberger N, Veroff J (eds): The Culture and Psychology Reader. New York, New York University Press, 1995. *Contains seminal chapters/articles on assessment, family, and therapy.*

Gordon J (ed): Managing Multiculturalism in Substance Abuse Services. Thousand Oaks, CA, Sage, 1996

Grinberg L, Grinberg R: Psychoanalytic Perspectives on Migration and Exile. New Haven, CT, Yale University Press, 1989

Group for the Advancement of Psychiatry: Alcoholism in the United States: Racial and Ethnic Considerations. Washington, DC, American Psychiatric Press, 1996

Harris HW, Blue HC, Griffith EEH (eds): Racial and Ethnic Identity. New York, Routledge, 1995

**Helms JE, Cook DA: Using Race and Culture in Counseling and Psychotherapy: Theory and Process. Boston, MA, Allyn and Bacon, 1999. *An outstanding textbook on racial and cultural themes in psychotherapy.*

Hernandez M, Isaacs MR: Promoting Cultural Competence in Children's Mental Health Services. Baltimore, MD, Paul H Brookes, 1998. *An essential guide to cultural competence in this area.*

Hood R, Spilka B, Hunsberger B, et al: The Psychology of Religion, 2nd Edition. New York, Guilford, 1996

Jackson LC, Greene B (eds): Psychotherapy With African American Women. New York, Guilford, 2000

Jaranson J, Popkin M (eds): Caring for Victims of Torture. Washington, DC, American Psychiatric Press, 1998

**Johnson-Powell G, Yamamoto J (eds): Transcultural Child Development: Psychological Assessment and Treatment. New York, Wiley, 1997. *Comprehensive overview of human development from a cultural perspective.*

Jones J: Prejudice and Racism, 2nd Edition. New York, McGraw Hill, 1997. *Outstanding historical and sociological perspectives.*

**Kleinman A: Rethinking Psychiatry. New York, Free Press, 1988. *The most important conceptual work in cross-cultural psychiatry—a classic.*

*Larson DB, Lu FG, Swyers JP (eds): Model Curriculum for Psychiatry Residency Training Programs: Religion and Spirituality in Clinical Practice. Rockville, MD, National Institute for Healthcare Research, 1996. *Very important for those planning curriculum in this area.*

Larson DB, Swyers JP, McCullough ME (eds): Scientific Research on Spirituality and Health: A Consensus Report. Rockville, MD, National Institute for Healthcare Research, 1998. *An extraordinary synthesis of the research literature.*

*Lee E (ed): Working With Asian Americans. New York, Guilford, 1997. *An important comprehensive, clinically oriented text.*

Lee LC, Zane NWS (eds): Handbook of Asian American Psychology. Thousand Oaks, CA, Sage, 1998

Leininger M: Transcultural Nursing. New York, McGraw-Hill, 1995

*Lin K-M, Poland RE, Nakasaki G, et al (eds): Psychopharmacology and Psychobiology of Ethnicity. Washington, DC, American Psychiatric Press, 1993. *The definitive work in this area.*

Lipson JG, Steiger NJ: Self-Care Nursing in a Multicultural Context. Thousand Oaks, CA, Sage, 1996

*Lipson JG, Dibble SL, Minarik PA (eds): Culture Nursing Care: A Pocket Guide. San Francisco, CA, UCSF Nursing Press, 1996. *Essential for those providing nursing care of culturally diverse patients.*

Locke D: Improving Multicultural Understanding, 2nd Edition. Thousand Oaks, CA, Sage, 1998

Marsella AJ, Friedman MJ, Gerrity ET, et al (eds): Ethnocultural Aspects of Posttraumatic Stress Disorder: Issues, Research, and Clinical Applications. Washington, DC, American Psychological Association, 1996. *Essential overview for those working in this area.*

*McGoldrick M (ed): Re-Visioning Family Therapy: Race, Culture, and Gender in Clinical Practice. New York, Guilford, 1998

**McGoldrick M, Giordano J, Pearce J (eds): Ethnicity and Family Therapy, 2nd Edition. New York, Guilford, 1996. *Outstanding, comprehensive review of cultures and family systems.*

Mezzich J, Kleinman A, Fabrega H, et al (eds): Culture and Psychiatric Diagnosis: A DSM-IV Perspective. Washington, DC, American Psychiatric Press, 1996. *Articles from the National Institute of Mental Health Workgroup on Culture, Diagnosis, and Care submitted to the American Psychiatric Association Task Force on DSM-IV.*

Miller WR (ed): Integrating Spirituality Into Treatment. Washington, DC, American Psychological Association, 1999. *Well researched and practical.*

*New York State Office of Mental Health: Cultural Competence Performance Measures for Managed Behavioral Healthcare Programs. Albany, NY, New York State Office of Mental Health, 1998. *Essential for understanding systems cultural competence.*

Okpaku SO (ed): Clinical Methods in Transcultural Psychiatry. Washington, DC, American Psychiatric Press, 1998

Paniagua F: Assessing and Treating Culturally Diverse Individuals, 2nd Edition. Thousand Oaks, CA, Sage, 1998

Pargament K: The Psychology of Religion and Coping. New York, Guilford, 1997

**Pedersen P, Draguns J, Lonner W, et al (eds): Counseling Across Cultures, 4th Edition. Thousand Oaks, CA, Sage, 1996. *Cutting-edge chapters from a counseling psychology perspective.*

**Pinderhughes E: Understanding Race, Ethnicity, and Power. New York, Free Press, 1988. *A classic on the impact of race, ethnicity, and power on the interpersonal dynamics in therapy. Experientially focused.*

Ponterotto J, Pedersen P: Preventing Prejudice. Thousand Oaks, CA, Sage, 1993

**Ponterotto JJ, Casas Suzuki L, Alexander C (eds): Handbook of Multicultural Counseling. Thousand Oaks, CA, Sage, 1995. *The standard textbook. Very comprehensive.*

*Pope-Davis DB, Coleman HLK (eds): Multicultural Counseling Competencies: Assessment, Education and Training, and Supervision. Thousand Oaks, CA, Sage, 1996

**Richards PS, Bergin AE: A Spiritual Strategy for Counseling and Psychotherapy. Washington, DC, American Psychological Association, 1997. *Extraordinary synthesis on the psychotherapy-spirituality interface.*

Richards PS, Bergin AE: Handbook of Psychotherapy and Religious Diversity. Washington, DC, American Psychological Association, 2000

**Ridley C: Overcoming Unintentional Racism in Counseling and Therapy. Thousand Oaks, CA, Sage, 1995. *Essential reading on an extraordinarily difficult topic.*

Roysircar-Sodowsky G, Impara RC (eds): Multicultural Assessment in Counseling and Clinical Psychology. Lincoln, NE, University of Nebraska, 1996

*Ruiz P (ed): Cross-cultural psychiatry, in American Psychiatric Press Review of Psychiatry, Vol 14. Edited by Oldham J, Riba M. Washington, DC, American Psychiatric Press, 1995. *Concise chapters on assessment, psychotherapy, and psychopharmacology.*

**Ruiz P (ed): Ethnicity and Psychopharmacology (Review of Psychiatry, Vol 19). Washington, DC, American Psychiatric Press, 2000. *An update of Lin 1993.*

Samuda RJ: Psychological Testing of American Minorities: Issues and Consequences, 2nd Edition. Thousand Oaks, CA, Sage, 1998

*Scotton B, Chinen A, Battista J (eds): Textbook of Transpersonal Psychiatry and Psychology. New York, Basic Books, 1996. *Essential reading for those interested in spirituality and psychiatry.*

*Shafranske E (ed): Religion and the Clinical Practice of Psychology. Washington, DC, American Psychological Association, 1996. *Best-selling comprehensive overview.*

*Sue D, Sue D: Counseling the Culturally Different, 3rd Edition. New York, Wiley, 1999. *An update on a classic from counseling psychology.*

*Sue D, Ivey A, Pedersen P (eds): A Theory of Multicultural Counseling and Therapy. Pacific Grove, CA, Brooks/Cole, 1996. *Analogous in scholarly importance to counseling psychology as Rethinking Psychiatry is for psychiatry.*

*Sue DW, Carter RT, Casas JM, et al: Multicultural Counseling Competencies. Thousand Oaks, CA, Sage, 1998

Suzuki LA, Meller PJ, Ponterotto JG (eds): Handbook of Multicultural Assessment. San Francisco, CA, Jossey-Bass, 1996

Thompson C, Carter R (eds): Racial Identity Theory. Mahvah, NJ, Erlbaum, 1997

Ting-Toomey S: Communicating Across Cultures. New York, Guilford, 1999

Tseng W-S, Streltzer J (eds): Culture and Psychopathology: A Guide to Clinical Assessment. New York, Brunner/Mazel, 1997

Tseng W-S, Streltzer J (eds): Culture and Psychotherapy: A Guide to Clinical Practice. Washington, DC, American Psychiatric Press, 2001

Young-Bruehl E: The Anatomy of Prejudices. Cambridge, MA, Harvard University Press, 1996. *A psychoanalytic perspective on many forms of prejudice. Very scholarly.*

*Westermeyer JJ: Psychiatric Care of Migrants: A Clinical Guide. Washington, DC, American Psychiatric Press, 1989. *A practical guide. Very useful in clinical care.*

Appendix C

GLOSSARY OF CULTURAL PSYCHIATRY TERMS

Alloplastic   An approach in psychotherapy with the goal of effecting changes in the external environment. (see also *autoplastic*)

Autoplastic   An approach in psychotherapy with the goal of changing oneself to accommodate the external circumstances. (see also *alloplastic*)

Credibility   One of two basic elements (see also *giving*) introduced by psychologists Stanley Sue and Nolan Zane for appropriate application of cultural knowledge that are linked to particular processes that result in effective intercultural psychotherapy. Credibility refers to the client's perception of the therapist as an effective and trustworthy helper.

Cross-cultural psychopharmacology   The special area of pharmacology that deals with the variation in psychotropic drug responses in different populations and the contribution of pharmacological factors to such variations.

Culture   Meanings, values, and behavioral norms that are learned and transmitted in the dominant society and within its social groups. Culture powerfully influences cognitions, feelings, and the "self" concept, as well as the diagnostic process and treatment decisions (DSM-IV). Culture is a set of standards for behavior that a group of people attribute to those around them and that they use to orient their behavior (Goodenough).

Culture-bound syndrome Recurrent, locality-specific patterns of aberrant behavior and troubling experiences, indigenously considered to be "illness" or at least affliction, generally limited to specific societies or culture areas. These are localized, folk diagnostic categories that frame coherent meanings for certain repetitive, patterned, and troubling sets of experiences and observations. These include named categories in folk nosological systems, as well as "idioms of distress," or culturally salient expressions for communicating symptoms (DSM-IV).

Demoralization hypothesis Introduced by Jerome Frank, M.D., to explain how psychotherapy works. It posits that patients, whatever their symptoms, share a type of distress that responds to the components common to all schools of psychotherapy. Demoralization suggests a state of mind characterized by one or more of the following: subjective incompetence, loss of self-esteem, alienation, hopelessness (feeling that no one can help), or helplessness (feeling that other people could help but will not). Demoralization is thought to manifest itself through subjective symptoms (anxiety, depression, loneliness) or behavioral disturbance (interpersonal conflicts). Frank suggests that improvement resulting from psychotherapy lies in its ability to restore the patient's morale, with the consequent diminution or disappearance of symptoms.

Emic Derived from *phonemic*. One of two (see also *etic*) contrasting levels of data or methods of analysis introduced by Kenneth L. Pike that explains the ideology or behavior of members of a culture according to indigenous definitions. Emic models are culture-specific.

Ethnicity Collectivity of people within a larger society defined on the basis of both common origins, shared symbols, and standards for behavior (Schermerhorn).

Etic Derived from *phonetic*. One of two (see also *emic*) contrasting levels of data or models of analysis based on criteria from outside a particular culture. Etic models are held to be universal.

Expressive transaction The human interaction and rapport between the two persons in psychotherapy. Expressive transaction rests heavily on the personality attributes of the two individuals (Bloom and Summey). (see also *instrumental transaction*)

Extensive metabolizers Individuals with a normal amount of enzymes that participate in metabolic activities. (see also *poor metabolizers*)

Giving The patient's perception that something was received from the therapeutic encounter (Sue and Zane). (see also *credibility*)

Haan A Korean term that refers to an individual and collective subconscious emotional complex among Korean people, involving suppressed feelings of anger, rage, despair, frustration, holding grudges, indignation, and revenge. It is a syndrome believed to result from victimization of a Korean person both as an individual and as a Korean and is thought to be an important factor in the development of *hwa-byung* (anger disease). (see also *hwa-byung* in Appendix A, Glossary of Culture-Bound Syndromes in DSM-IV)

Inducers Substrates that increase the synthesis of P450 enzymes and have the effect of increasing the rate of biotransformation and reducing the serum level of the parent compound.

Inhibitors Substrates that decrease the synthesis of P450 enzymes and that usually result from competition between two or more drugs for the active site of the same enzyme. The resulting effects are an increased serum level of the less-metabolized parent compound, prolonged pharmacological effect, and increased incidences of drug-induced toxicities.

Instrumental transaction The special knowledge, skills, and procedures imparted in the process of healing between the two persons in psychotherapy (Bloom and Summey). (see also *expressive transaction*)

Monooxygenases   Hepatic cytochrome P450 isoenzymes located at the smooth endoplasmic reticulum of the liver and found to catalyze the oxidative reaction in phase I metabolism of most drugs.

Operating culture   Standards a person used at a particular time with significant others.

Operating procedure   Ways in which people organize their effort to accomplish certain purposes.

Pharmacodynamics   The biochemical and physiological effects of drugs at their loci of actions in the body.

Pharmacogenetics   The special area of biochemical genetics that deals with variation in drug response and the contribution of genetics to such variation.

Pharmacokinetics   The general bodily response to the presence of xenobiotics (such as drugs) in the human body. Phamacokinetics is the study of the biochemical and physiological processes involved in the process of absorption, distribution, metabolism (biotransformation), and excretion of a drug that determines its final plasma concentration.

Polymorphism   The condition in pharmacogenetics when two or more alternative genotypes are present in a population, each at a frequency greater than that which could be maintained by recurrent mutation alone; it is reflected in a bimodal or trimodal distribution of the activity of a drug-metabolizing enzyme (Thompson). Polymorphism may result in deficient or impaired enzymatic activities.

Poor metabolizers   Individuals with enzymatic mutation(s) resulting in deficient enzymatic activities. (see also *extensive metabolizers*)

Proletarianization   McKinney used this term to denote the process by which any occupational category is divested of control over certain prerogatives relating to the location, content, and essentiality of its task activities and is thereby subordinated to the broader requirements of production under advanced capitalism.

Psychotherapy A planned, emotionally charged, confiding interaction between a trained, socially sanctioned healer and a sufferer (Frank).

Race A number of broad divisions of the human species into groups, based on a common geographic origin, certain shared physical characteristics, and a characteristic distribution of gene frequencies.

Spirit Dance A Native American ceremonial dance of the Coast Salish Indians that has been employed to treat the problem of alcoholism among Indians. Both the Spirit Dance and the Sioux Sun Dance focus on individual autonomy, strong kinship ties, community unification and affirmation of ancestral continuity, and guidelines and alternatives for behavior. The Spirit Dance requires abstinence from alcohol and drugs for an extended period of time.

Subculture Narrower sets of standards that govern how one acts within a smaller range of behavior with a particular set of actors.

Sweat A Native American healing ritual performed by pouring water over hot rocks, which produces steam for purposes of prayers, cleansing, and healing.

System The concept that refers to both the complex of interdependencies between parts, components, and processes that involves discernible regularities of relationship, and to a similar type of interdependency between such a complex and the surrounding environment (Parson).

Windigo An Algonkian Indian's idiom of distress often associated with the idea of the mystery and great concerns over a lost person. Windigo is often cited in the literature as referring to the idea of cannibal compulsion among Algonkian Indians.

INDEX

*Page numbers printed in **boldface** refer to tables or figures.*